Stretching on the Pilates Reformer
Essential Cues and Images

Anthony Lett / Kenyi Diaz

First published July 2016
Text © Innovations in Pilates, 2016
Published by Innovations in Pilates
with the assistance of Rebus Press
Innovations in Pilates
1 Regina St. Rosanna
VIC 3085 Australia
www.innovationsinpilates.com
Rebus Press
PO Box 622
Hurstbridge VIC 3099
Email: julie@rebuspress.com.au
Web: www.rebuspress.com.au
Anatomy diagrams used with permission of Muscle and Motion
Cover design by Kenyi Diaz
Layout by Kenyi Diaz
Modelling by Kenyi Diaz, Anthony Lett

National Library of Australia Cataloguing-in-Publication entry

Creator:	Lett, Anthony, author.
Title:	Innovations in pilates : matwork for health and wellbeing / Anthony Lett, Kenyi Diaz.
ISBN:	978-0-9945147-1-4 (paperback)
Subjects:	Pilates method.
	Health.
	Physical fitness.
Other Creators/ Contributors:	Diaz, Kenyi, author.
Dewey Number:	613.7192

Graphic Images
An enormous thanks to our very talented medical/anatomical animator/designer Amit Gal Anon. Amit has a very special story to tell, and creates his own fabulous range of anatomy software. Check it out at www.muscleandmotion.com

Special thanks to Angela Shi. A fabulously creative designer who did a lot of work with Kenyi preparing the final layout. Moreover, Angie is the ONLY prompt, efficient, deadline observing graphic designer I have ever met (not including Kenyi of course!) Thank you! You can contact Angie through www.cargocollective.com/angebots.

Special Thanks to I.C Rapoport who provided one of the fabulous images he took of Joe Pilates back in 1961 as a photojournalist for Sports Illustrated. You can read about it at http://icrapoport.com/a-day-with-joseph-pilates/

Photography by another talented artist and award winning photographer Ady Lander. Based in Collingwood Melbourne, Ady is a delight to work with and an elite Pilates practitioner too! http://filmbyalf.com/about-film-by-alf/

Editing
Thanks again to Julie Jay from Rebus Press. Laid back, reliable, and smart. A terrific trio of qualities.

Anthony

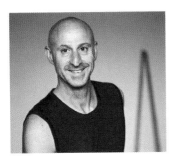

... is a Pilates studio owner, teacher, educator and writer originally from Melbourne Australia. Anthony teaches workshops globally on the material from his books titled *Innovations in Pilates*. Anthony is the Director of Advanced Education for BASI Pilates and has qualifications in philosophy, sports science, exercise medicine and clinical anatomy. Anthony has presented his workshops and keynote addresses in over 25 countries and is a leading creative thinker in the Pilates industry. Anthony's three books contain fascinating world-first 3D Pilates graphics and merge practices from osteopathy, physiotherapy and Yoga with traditional Pilates repertoire. A fourth, titled *On Pilates* is on the way. Anthony also created the first *Pilates Anatomy* certification course, as well as the first 3D printed Pilates reformer. *Pilates Anatomy* involves three-dimensional anatomy video, creation of muscles on skeletons, and exploration of functional anatomy in the Pilates studio. Anthony and his wife, Kenyi, run a small studio on the Panama Canal and teach retreats in Bali Indonesia.

anthony@innovationsinpilates.com
http://anthonylett.com.au/
www.innovationsinpilates.com

Kenyi

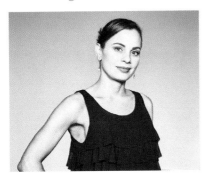

... is a professional Pilates instructor originally from Venezuela, with a background in dance, and training in classical and contemporary Pilates. Kenyi began teaching Pilates in 2004. Kenyi has taught Innovations in Pilates workshops in Australia, Asia, Europe, the UK, South Africa and South America. A skilled graphic artist, Kenyi designed and co-authored all of the *Innovations in Pilates* materials including books, ebooks and video production. Kenyi is pursuing an academic interest in human nutrition; in particular, eating for health and wellbeing, for sports performance, and in the growing area of "food as medicine".

kenyi@innovationsinpilates.com
www.kenyidiaz.com
www.innovationsinpilates.com

Contents

Preface

The quote above is the basis for this book. Simple cues and powerful images convey what can be complex biomechanical relationships in the simplest manner possible. While my first book in the series – titled *Innovations in Pilates, Therapeutic Muscle Stretching on the Pilates Reformer* – was, dare I say it, a more cerebral approach, this book is a visual version. Is it a dumbed down approach? I don't think so. It represents certain realities. One is a recognition of how people learn. I call it the "IKEA test". Have you ever assembled IKEA furniture? Did you carefully read the instruction manual before making a start, or did you look at the images and take it from there? If you read everything first, you probably fall into the cerebral camp.

If you relied on the images, your brain might be wired a little differently, and this book is for you. For true mastery (and for your IKEA wardrobe to stay upright), the best approach is to do both. But, as stretching, bodywork and personal development is a complicated and non-linear process, start at the place that feels more accessible and 'right' for you.

The second reason for this book is that the first reformer book was a way, for me, of clarifying through writing what I thought I knew. Six years and hundreds of workshops, presentations and classes later, I know much more, and presenting information in a different style makes sense to me now.

Another reality is that not everyone wants to read a treatise on stretching. This became clear to me after teaching workshops around the world for the past five years, based on the material in the first book. Many people had simply not read it! So what is the skilful option? Force them to read something that doesn't meet their learning style, has more depth than what they want or are ready for? Or take a different route and provide information in what is, for some, a more palatable form? With this book, I offer the latter. Enjoy the compressed, need to know, visual approach. This is the "taste the food, read the recipe later" approach.

A note on the historical images. The very old pictures I've included of Joseph Pilates and his wife, Clara, allow you to travel back in time and witness some of the original material. You will see the antecedents to some of the Innovations material. Although the quality is not always good, they will connect you to Joe Pilates and may give you some insights into his personality and his story.

Introduction
Part A

In case you haven't noticed, this book is about how to increase your flexibility, range of movement (ROM) or suppleness. While we could split hairs about definitions, to me these are all essentially the same thing. In any case, we all understand what stretching is in a practical sense, and I prefer to split muscles and fascia. In fact, the more perplexing questions seem to be, "What is stretching good for?" and ,"Which method is best to enhance range of movement?"

In my reformer book I provide a multitude of reasons as to the benefits of stretching. The list is long and can be viewed from different perspectives: physical, psychological, biological, biomechanical, neural, hormonal, immunological, athletic, spiritual[1]. And new research keeps growing the list. In the spirit of keeping this book simple, let's just say stretching has huge benefits. (Readers who are curious can follow up some references at the end of the book).

One of my favourite expressions is "aerobic exercise will keep you alive, while stretching will make it worth being alive". You could substitute strength training for aerobic training too, I think. Stretching will improve the quality of your life, not just the quantity. The fundamental movement patterns of our lives, like bending, squatting, pulling, pushing, twisting, turning and reaching, can all be maintained, and in fact improved as we age, with the work inside this book. Although I have not yet reached old age, I am confident that, as I do, the ability to get around and to do so relatively pain free will undoubtedly make me happier to be alive. So invest some trust in the following practices (tested over a 15 year period in my studio on many thousands of clients) and in the research that exists to bring about some very significant benefits to your life.

(1) Footnote: Many of the books listed at the completion of the book will provide strong arguments for the practice of stretching. I want to raise just two issues.

The first is that we should not confine our discussion only to biomechanics. The field of mind–body medicine now provides a huge amount of research and data to support such practices as stillness, breathing, yoga, meditation and stretching in effectively countering the effects of chronic stress.

The *World Health Organization* attributes 70% to 80% of visits to medical practitioners in the first world to the effects of stress. So although stretching will help to counterbalance biomechanical stress on the muscles and joints of the body, it has a much larger role to play. For further information on this subject, a good place to start is Herbert Benson's book, *The Relaxation Response*.

The second issue to raise is that many discussions in the popular press around stretching relate to the efficacy of stretching for sporting performance. Specifically, does stretching improve performance and reduce injury? Again, there is a huge amount of data to support stretching on both counts.

One problem with this question is that it needs to be explored with some depth...and depth is not something for which the popular media is noted. Also, one needs to know something about the validity of the research. And finally, one needs to question the question itself.

Does it matter if stretching improves sporting perfomance? After all, most people over the age of 25 don't play any sport. Isn't it more important to ascertain if stretching can improve the quality of one's life into old age? Despite difficulties in measuring this outcome, we know that it does.

Do we constantly ask if aerobic exercise improves sporting performance? Of course, for some sports we know that it does; but the question is irrelevant to the millions who jog, cycle, swim and do Zumba, either for fun or for the benefits to their overall health, irrespective of whether it improves performance in any of competitive sporting arena.

Why Innovations in Pilates?

"Constantly keep in mind that
you are not interested in merely
developing bulging muscles but
rather, flexible ones."
-Joe Pilates, *Your Health*

A detailed history of *Innovations in Pilates*
and its development can be found in my
previous reformer book. For now, permit me
to give you some insights.

Joe Pilates had a strong interest in the
acquisition of flexibility, yet interest in this
aspect of his work was starting to wane.
We didn't want to see this happen. Why?
Because flexibility is an important human
attribute, and as a quality its practice is more
important in today's sedentary digital world
than ever before.

Flexibility is also an essential tenet of
the Pilates method; worth preserving for
this reason alone. Moreover, much of the
traditional repertoire requires considerable
flexibility to perform. In this respect,
Innovations in Pilates can be seen as a form
of pre-Pilates for stiff people who want to
take up the method. It can also function as
preparation for the more advanced repertoire
if that is your interest.

According
to Joseph Pilates' original
protégé, Romana Kryzanowska,
when asked, "What is contrology?" (the
name he gave to his method) Joe would
reply, "It is stretch, with strength and control."
In his book titled *Your Health*, Pilates wrote:
"Contrology was conceived to limber and
stretch muscles so that you will be as
supple as a cat."

To continue this theme we offer
you *Innovations in Pilates*.

So what have we done in creating Innovations in Pilates?

Many of the original exercises are too difficult and potentially unsafe for today's sedentary population …

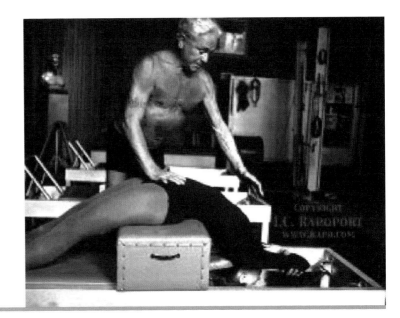

.. so we have introduced a range of contemporary modifications and variations.

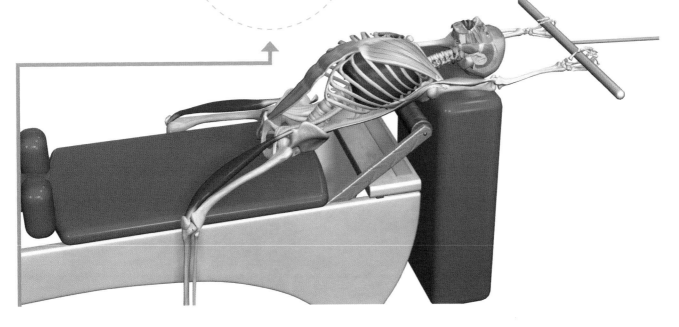

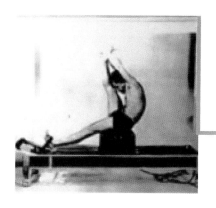

We included some modern neuromuscular techniques from physiotherapy and sports science to improve outcomes. We call it "classical origins, contemporary infusions' (technical details later).

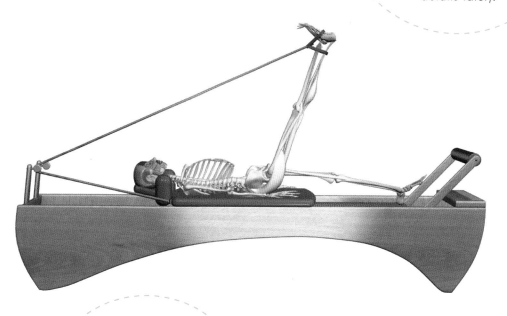

"Perform an isometric contraction by pushing both feet into the reformer for 5 seconds, then relax, restretch and hold for 60 to 90 seconds".

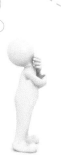

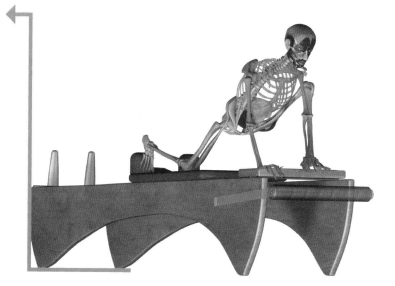

We've
slowed down the
stretches to avoid triggering
reflexive responses from
your nervous system that
work against optimal
outcomes.

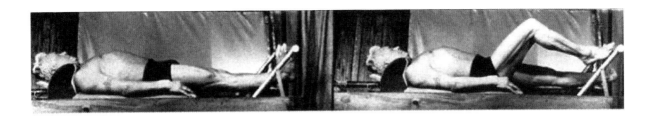

"Instead
of performing this
at speed, like Joe above,
lower one heel and hold for 90
seconds. Research suggests this
is safer and more effective
for flexibility gains".

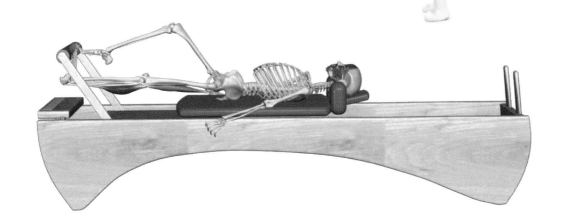

We've added a few new stretches where none existed.

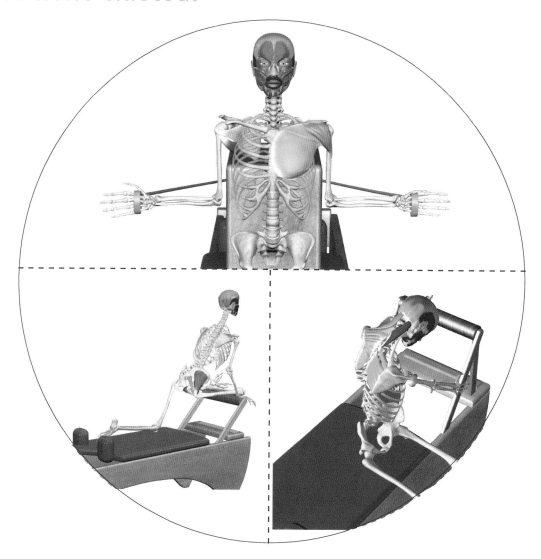

The end result...

Practising the work in this book will prepare you for the more advanced Pilates repertoire, if that is your interest.

As a teacher, it will allow you to re-introduce or increase the stretching element of Pilates and work in a safe and effective manner.

Whether your interest is to improve sporting performance or simply to improve your range of movement, rid yourself of aches and pains, and move with more grace and ease in life, I know of no better way to achieve it. If there were one, we would readily embrace it!

Part B

Getting it right

"Don't teach scripts, teach understanding; so that you or your students can write their own scripts — their understanding which they own."
-Anthony Lett

As a teacher and student most of my life, I have come to believe that, particularly in the learning of physical skills, the old model of "right and wrong" where the infallible teacher doles out verbal corrections and physical adjustments is flawed.

What students require is not to be spoon fed facts or instructions. In fact, too much information can get in the way. What students respond to, particularly in the learning of physical skills like stretching, is a teacher who facilitates self-enquiry. Students asking questions and being encouraged to feel what's happening inside of themselves is far more effective than listening to the teacher reporting what they see from the outside.

This type of teaching makes the student less dependent on others, providing an external frame of reference. In time, students develop embodied understanding, which they hold with confidence and become their own teachers.

But how do we balance this model of learning alongside the perfect photographs and anatomical images in this book? We can do this by drawing a distinction between the aesthetic (how something looks) and the kinesthetic/experiential (how something feels). The aesthetic is how we make a start. Take a look at the photos, read the scripts and try to emulate or engage in them. This gives us a frame of reference, a place to begin and ensures that we are quite likely to feel the stretch in roughly the right places.

Then, turn to the kinesthetic–experiential dimension. How does it feel? Where are the feelings coming from? These are the more critical questions; far more important than how closely you resemble the model in the photograph. Ask yourself these questions in your practice. This form of inquiry will greatly extend the breadth of your practice. You may find that, yes, your hamstrings are tight, but that there are also feelings and sensations from other areas worth investigating.

It may be helpful to add here that no feelings during a stretch are 'wrong'. Some people may 'feel it', while others won't be sure but will try to convince themselves they're feeling it. Some people will feel something else and wonder what they're doing wrong, and some people will have the experience of, "I don't know what the hell I'm feeling!"

This is all okay and normal, and needs to be understood. Desikachar, one of the originators of therapeutic yoga, would often say that the recognition of confusion itself is a form of clarity, and that (all) knowledge begins with that recognition.

A note to teachers: Frequent corrections aren't without risk. They can leave students with the impression that they need fixing, that there's something wrong with their bodies or lacking in their abilities. The truth is that no two bodies are the same. To put it another way, no one's One leg dog pose will look exactly like anyone else's. There is no single normal.

Each of your students and their bodies are a unique mix of psychosocial, biochemical and biomechanical influences. They appear before you as a personal adaptive configuration of these influences superimposed on their unique inherited characteristics. These are the differences that you have to work with.

Let's not forget too that out in the world we are bombarded with images of perfection, and that we do not need to perpetuate this in our practice. It leads to a kind of "judgmentalness", another set of standards against which we can fail. Stretching work is at least as much about the inner work as the outer form. Let's not obsess about the angle of that knee!

As my father has always taught in his work as a professor and practitioner of psychotherapy, "Recognition of felt knowing always makes a contribution of value to our understanding." I am sure this applies in the current context also.

Descriptions of movement

Throughout this text, you will hear descriptions of movements like 'hip flexion', 'abduction', 'external rotation' et cetera. Typically, in most books there will be a figure at around this section demonstrating planes of movement. I have decided against this feature because I think, in this book in particular, you will learn to make sense of the language of movement in the process of moving.

Experience, as we all know, is the best of teachers. Use the many diagrams, internal inquiry, our videos and online workshops where necessary, and a good teacher to refine your work. You will learn more meaningfully about moving by moving.

The Pilates reformer

Joseph Pilates designed many pieces of equipment. For readers with an historical interest the official name of the reformer was the 'universal reformer'. His vison was that everyone, everywhere, would use one. The reformer was not designed solely for stretching, but as stretching tools go I have never used anything even remotely as good. It is my hope to continue Joe's vision of universality in the sense that I hope that everyone, everywhere, will take up the life changing practice of stretching.

A note on standards (which stretches should you do?)

Flexibility is joint specific. Few people are stiff everywhere. Even fewer are flexible everywhere. With this in mind, generalising stretches as 'beginner', 'intermediate' or 'advanced' is not unproblematic. Sometimes, for example, 'advanced' implies a degree of flexibility required to enable you to make a start.

Other times it may imply a degree of strength, balance and body awareness as a prerequisite. What you will probably find is that in some regions you are stiff, in others you are not. You may also intuit this by looking at the images.

Whatever the case, I encourage you to explore all of the material with awareness. Investigate yourself. Self-observation and internal inquiry is an incredibly useful skill, with benefits far beyond the acquisition of flexibility. Locate your tight areas and work at them. Said Mr Pilates, **"Study your body – know it's good and bad points. Eliminate the bad and improve the good."** (*Your Health*, p.25).

How often should I stretch?

"A few well-designed movements, properly performed, are worth hours of doing sloppy calisthenics or forced contortion."
-Joseph Pilates

I have written more extensively about this in our previous two books. However, the question does allow me to regurgitate one of my favourite quotations from Sartre. Sartre observed, **"We are the authors of ourselves, through our actions, and our failures to act, we ultimately design ourselves".** In a physical sense, all of our behaviour stimulates adaptation.

We are constantly designing ourselves, for better or for worse. If we do very little exercise, for example, we lose muscle mass. Our bodies decide that muscle, which is metabolically and energetically very costly, is unnecessary; so we shed some of it.

Recent findings show similar adaptations in the brain. As we age, grey matter diminishes if it is not consistently challenged. Although these examples show negative adaptations, they are, nevertheless, response to stimuli or the lack there of.

Similarly, repeated exposure to stretching will drive another form of adaptation described as "mechanotransduction" (Lederman: Therapeutic Stretching). Mechanotransduction is the biological response of your tissues as they grow longer in response to the mechanical tensile stress they experience from stretching.

For mechanotransduction to occur, you must stretch each muscle group at least twice weekly. (Don't forget the other stimuli that you are unconsciously exposing yourself to, and battling against, like sitting in a chair). You must also hold the stretches for the length of time we have recommended.

Ylinen, in his book Stretching Therapy, details studies between groups that stretched for different periods of time (p.73). The group that held stretches for one minute had a 15% improvement in flexibility in just one month. The group that held stretches for 15 seconds improved just 4%. To me, 4% is not a worthwhile return on investment.

Bottom line: work thoroughly, follow our prescriptions and don't take shortcuts.

Spring tension

The recommendations that I have provided on spring tension selection are, admittedly, vague. There are several reasons for this. First, spring tension varies from brand to brand, and even between reformers of the same brand. In addition, how much spring tension you need will depend on how heavy you are, how strong you are, how stiff you are, how far you can move the carriage initially in the stretch, and your position in relation to the reformer. Sometimes the reformer spring tension deepens a stretch by gently pulling the carriage back to its resting position.

Other times, it is counterbalancing almost exactly the tension in your muscles and providing support. In addition to reading and following the spring selection that is recommended, please work with great awareness, especially in your first attempts at any stretch, until you find the appropriate support to enable relaxation.

There should be no jerking or sudden movement, which would ruin the strategy of inducing relaxation in the affected musculature. There should be no struggle to hold the carriage in position either. As Joe Pilates would say, **"Not too little, not too much"**.

Part C

The biomechanics of stretching

Before we get into the biomechanics of stretching, let's first understand what we are talking about. *What is stretching? What is stiffness?*

Stretching places muscles and fascia in lengthened positions for prescribed periods of time. Force is applied to achieve this change in length. The amount of force is determined by the stiffness of the tissues. There are two types of stiffness. One is reflex mediated. This means it is controlled by our nervous system, and is dependent on the excitability of motor neurons. The other is called intrinsic stiffness. This is the stiffness of the tissue in the absence of any electromyographical reading.

Intrinsic stiffness refers to the viscoelastic quality of muscle-existing bonds between actin and myosin. This is the stiffness or extensibility of the meat itself, and, as a mechanical property, could be measured for example when under a general anaesthetic, where your muscles are almost totally lacking in tone. With repeated stretching over time, we affect both types of stiffness.

Research demonstrates that the meat itself becomes freer and grows longer too, albeit it microscopically. Via stretching, a process called 'mechanotransduction' occurs, where a mechanical stress (i.e. a stretch) stimulates a biological adaptation. The adaptation is to grow longer muscles. It is as if we add a link to our muscular chain. Research also suggests that muscle 'grows' shorter too if movement is limited. (It's that damn 'use it or lose it' principle at work!)

Reflexes are altered too. Your brain becomes rewired and new patterns and ranges of movement become possible without triggering reflexive pain signals.

Bottom line: Stretching is easy to define, and easy to practise. Stiffness is a little more complex. It has two types, one controlled by the central nervous system, the other independent of it.

What limits our flexibility?

Previously, we looked at muscle and fascia. We understand that they are alterable and to do so is safe. Shortly, we will look at the most effective way to do this. First though, let's look at what else can affect our flexibility.

The architecture of joints

This is a limiting factor for flexibility. Often, of course, stiffness will prevent you from discovering this because bones lock together long into a stretch and, usually, your muscles will stop you well short of this point. For some, though, unusual bony formation will prevent 'normal' ranges of motion. Because bone shape is permanent and cannot be changed once growth plates are closed (during adolescence), this limiting factor ought to be kept in mind. It has definitely prevented my own flexibility development, and knowledge of bony limitations could have prevented injury and countless hours of frustration for me.

If you feel a block somewhere into a stretch, and it is not a familiar stretching sensation, investigate the possibility of bone shape as its cause. Please read the section titled 'Tension and Compression' in our matbook *Innovations in Pilates, Matwork for Health and Wellbeing* for a more detailed discussion of this issue.

Image 1 gives some idea of the variation in bone shape. The overhanging acromion on the right will definitely limit what is known as 'normal' shoulder range of movement.

IMAGE 1

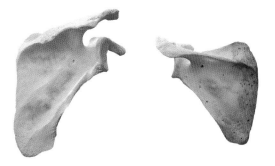

Capsuloligamentous structures

These also limit our flexibility. The joint capsule and ligaments are comprised of fibrous connective tissue which fasten bones to one another and provide joint stability and mobility.

Although capsuloligamentous structures vary depending on the joint, they have a limited capacity to stretch. To do so, although long lasting, would be painful, difficult and potentially destabilising.

IMAGE 2

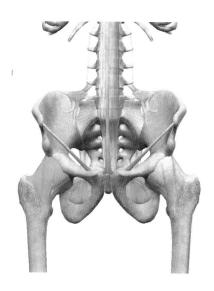

Image 2 is an example of the ligaments of the hip joint. Merging with the capsule, they limit end ranges of movement.

To stretch them, you would first have to overcome all muscular and neuromuscular limitations, potential strutural limitations, and tolerate a large amount of pain and force! As a result, they are, for 97% of the population who are not hypermobile, mostly irrelevant.

Bottom line: Although Capsuloligamentous structures can limit flexibility, unless you are hypermobile they are not particularly relevant for our practice.

Biomechanics of stretching

Since bone shape cannot be changed, and ligaments will not come to the party either, we are left to work with muscles and some types of fascia. Let's have a look at the basic biomechanics of stretching.

All muscles have an origin on one part of the skeleton and an insertion on another part. Stretching a muscle involves moving these two ends away from each other. Muscles can be stretched by anchoring one end and moving the other, or by moving both ends away from each other. Image 3 illustrates this concept.

The quadriceps contract to straighten the knee. This tightens one end of the hamstrings running across the back of the knee onto the lower leg. This end of the hamstrings is usually described as the insertion.

In addition, leaning forward to hold the bar and contracting the rectus femoris to straighten the leg pulls the pelvis toward the thigh bone or femur. This action, called hip flexion, moves the other end of the hamstrings (usually described as the origin) at the back of the pelvis on the sit bones, or ischial tuberosities, further from the insertion.

The result: the origin and insertion of the hamstrings are moved apart and you will experience this as the sensation of stretching.

Stretching physiology

When we stretch, as in the example above, receptors within joints, tendons and muscles detect movement and changes in muscle length and tension. These receptors alert the central nervous system (CNS) to this event for an appropriate response. If you stretch too fast, for example, your muscles will contract to prevent damage.

Aside from stretching, receptors alert your CNS to events such as jumping and landing, leaning, or touching something hot. Reflex signals travel to the spinal cord and back in what is called a reflex 'arc'. This enables a speedy response. It takes a second or two for messages to reach the brain itself – too long in this instance. Often, it is only after the reflex has occurred and the message arrives in the brain that you become aware of it.

We have a complex array of receptors and reflex arcs linking our muscles to our

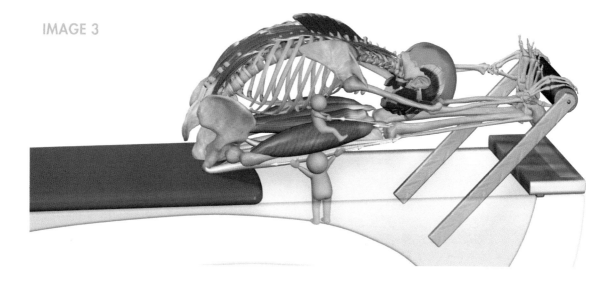

central nervous system. Two stretch receptors are most relevant to us. The muscle spindle stretch receptor detects changes in length and the speed of those changes. Basically, when a muscle stretches, the spindle sends a signal to the spinal cord, which then signals back to the to the muscle to contract and resist the stretch. This is known as the 'stretch reflex'.

Bottom line: Stretching at speed, like ballistic stretching, is counterproductive. It will fire the muscle spindle stretch receptor and cause the muscles to contract.

The Golgi tendon organ (GTO) is a different story altogether. This receptor organ, located where the muscle and tendon join, detects changes in muscle tension.

When tension increases, particularly if there is no limb movement, it signals muscles to relax to prevent injury. The GTO is like a thermostat, flicking off the heater to prevent a meltdown.

The GTO forms the basis of what is called the contract/relax (C/R) technique; just one of the many found in the body of work known as PNF or proprioceptive neuromuscular facilitation. We will use this C/R technique throughout this book to deepen and accelerate our flexibility progress.

Here's how it works:

1 Take yourself VERY SLOWLY into a mild stretch. We call this the POINT OF TENSION, or POT. Moving quickly will trigger the stretch reflex. On a scale of one to ten, one being not much of a stretch and ten being complete agony, we suggest a score of five or six. Hold the position for five breaths and settle.

2 Contract the muscles that you are trying to stretch. We will give you cues, of course; although it may seem counterintuitive, contract the muscles we recommend for five seconds. Use around 30 % of your maximum effort, and start gently.

3 Relax totally and restretch to the new position. Don't expect miracles, but you can expect to be able to go further into the stretch, often between 1 to 10 centimetres further. Hold the new POT for fifteen breaths.

Contract/relax in the posterior stretch

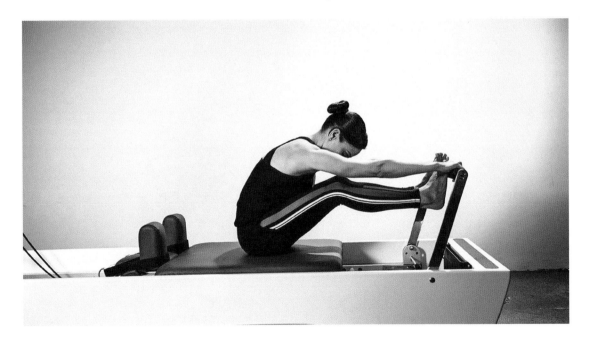

1 Press the carriage away to the POT. Hold for 5 breaths.

2 Contract the muscles you are stretching. In this case, it is the hamstrings. Contract for 5 seconds by pressing your feet down into the foot bar. Use 30% of maximum force. The GTO will signal increased tension via a sensory nerve to the spinal cord. A relaxation signal will travel to the muscle, facilitating a restretch.

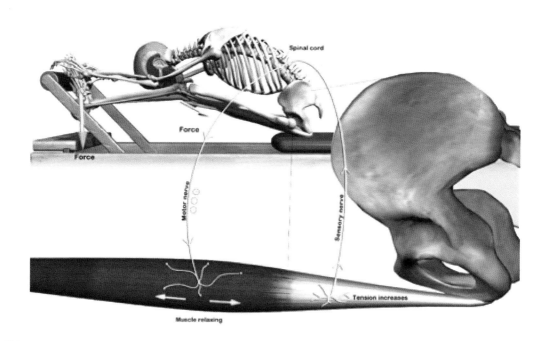

3 Relax and re-stretch to the new POT. Hold for 15 deep breaths. See image below.

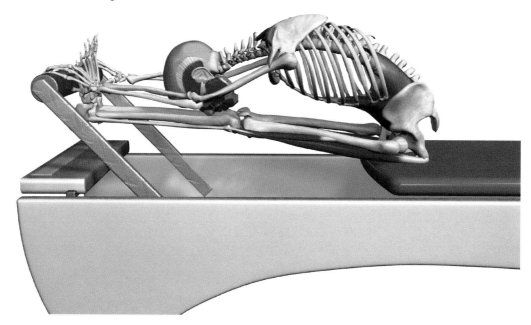

One final thing before you start

"How you do anything, is how you do everything."

I heard this astute observation just recently, and I like it. What does it mean? I think it means that whatever we are doing – be it stretching, drawing, writing, gardening, cooking, reading – we tend to do it in the same way that we do everything else. Do you rush too much? Are you self-critical, impatient, perfectionistic, lazy?

Often, life is so busy we don't even know the answer to these questions. Stretching will give you the time to take a look. Try it. The insight will be at least as beneficial as your gains in flexibility. Once you notice a trait, take that observation into the rest of your life.

The aim of his method, to quote Mr Pilates again, was to be, **"... fully capable of successfully meeting all the complex problems of modern living".** A little self-awareness won't hurt this pursuit.

Need to know from this chapter

There are various factors that assist and resist the pursuit of flexibility. If we work slowly, with awareness, we can make use of the positive and learn to feel, understand and occasionally accept the restrictive barriers as well. This will develop a peaceful and productive practice.

Chapter One

The Calves

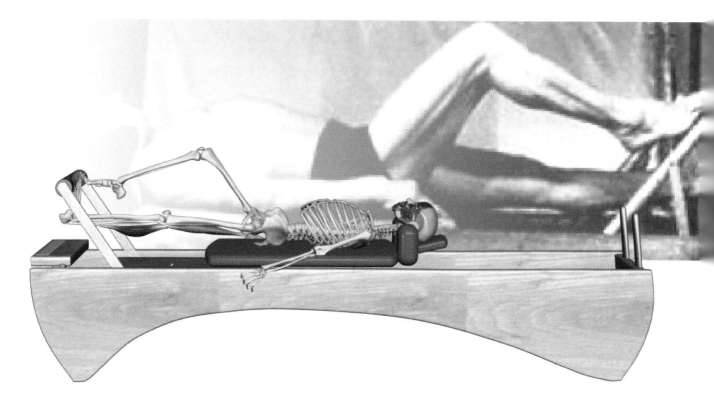

and lower leg compartments

The Lying Calves

- **Standard:** Any • **Spring Tension:** Medium - Heavy
- **Muscle Emphasis:** Entire calf group

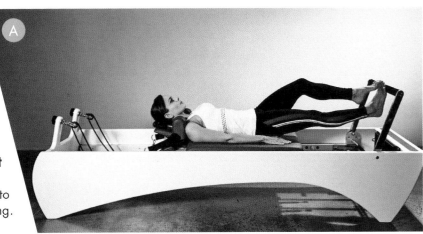

A. How to stretch

Press carriage away and lower one heel slowly to POT. Bend other knee. Tighten quadriceps in stretching leg.

A. How to contract

Press ball of foot that is stretching into foot bar as if accelerating.

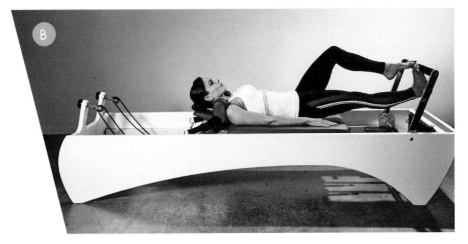

B & C. How to restretch

Lower heel slowly under bar.

What to watch out for:

- Gripping with toes
- Moving into stretch too quickly -"bouncing".
- Allowing knee to bend.

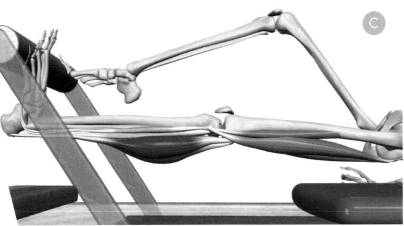

A partner can intensify this stretch in the gastrocnemius in particular by holding your heel and pulling it gently but firmly under the bar.

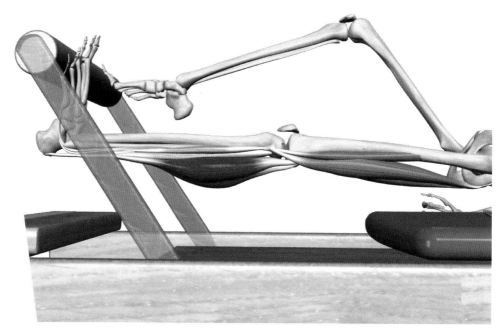

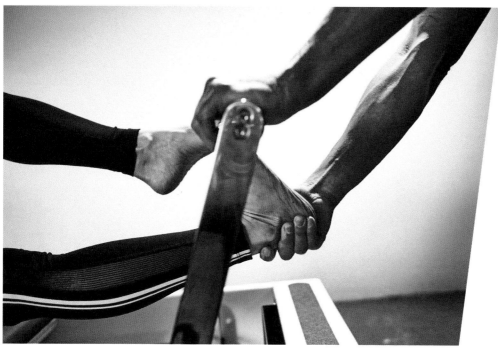

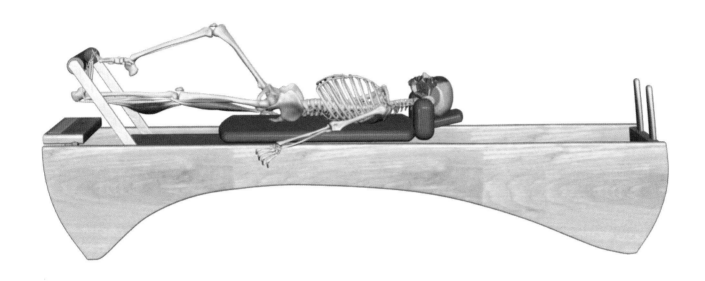

Underneath the gastrocnemius lies the soleus. Under the soleus are the flexors of the toes, flexors digitorum longus, flexor hallucis longus and tibialis posterior.

The Standing Calves

- **Standard:** Beginner - Intermediate • **Spring Tension:** Medium
- **Muscle Emphasis:** Entire calf group, hamstrings if tight!

A. How to stretch

Place heel against shoulder rest. Lift arch of foot. Place one foot behind the other. Keep hips level horizontally. Press carriage away to POT. Lean hips toward springs. Try to have shoulders/ arms roughly 90 degrees to chest.

A. How to contract

Press ball of foot down into carriage.

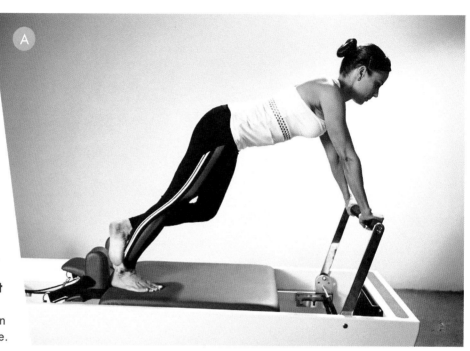

B. How to restretch

Press the carriage away a bit more, and lean hips toward foot bar.
Try to align shoulder, hip, ankle.

What to watch out for:

- Arch of foot collapsing.
- Knee bending.
- Hips rotating in a horizontal plane.

The Standing Calves 2.0

- **Standard:** Beginner - Intermediate • **Spring Tension:** Medium - Heavy
- **Muscle Emphasis:** Entire calf group, hamstrings, adductor magnus, gluteus maximus

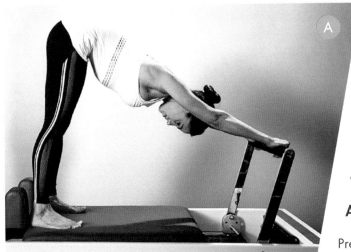

A. How to stretch

Press carriage away a little to POT as pictured, with both heels against shoulder rests. Lower chest to line up with arms if possible. Rotate pelvis anteriorly (forward) to point sit bones to ceiling. Lift chest to straighten spine.

A. How to contract

Press the balls of both feet down into carriage.

B & C. How to restretch

Bend one knee.
Slide carriage toward foot bar;
i.e. more hip flexion. Lower chest.
Arch spine backwards; i.e. straighten spine.

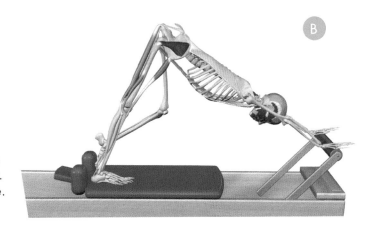

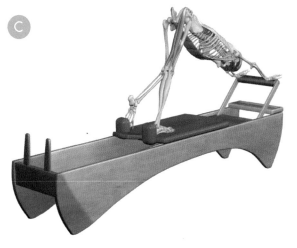

What to watch out for:

- Arches of feet collapsing.
- Knee that is stretching/bending.
- Pelvis rotating posteriorly.
- Spine rounding/flexing.
- Be sure to stretch both legs.

As the gastrocnemius is stretched with the hamstrings, the latissimus dorsi and rectus abdominus work strongly to stabilise and support the arms, shoulders and trunk.

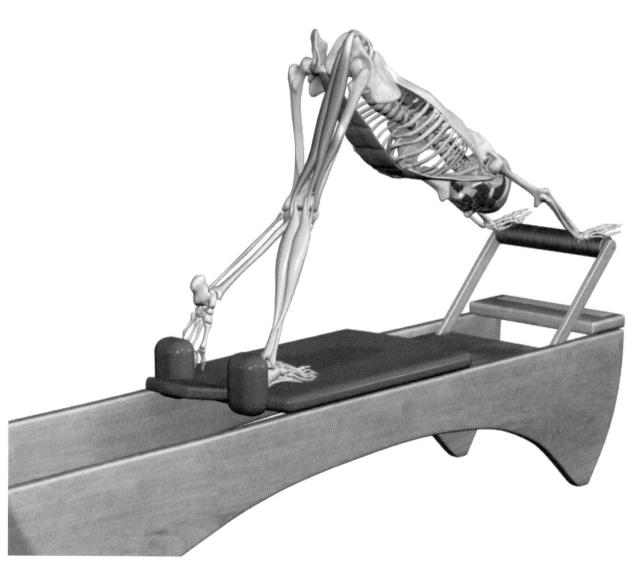

 To read about the work of the abdominals and lats in stabilising and supporting the spine, try our online workshop titled "Lengthening and Safeguarding the Spine in Forward Bending".

Variations

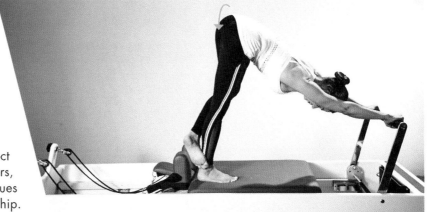

Raise hip of non-stance leg to affect medial hamstrings and adductors, quadratus lumborum and obliques on side of lifted hip.

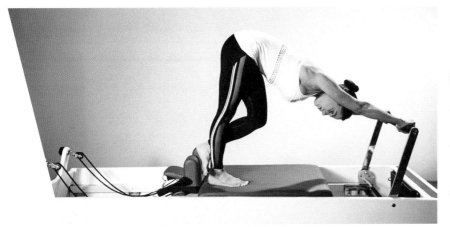

To read about the arch of the foot in this exercise, how to cue it, how to detect muscle imbalances, and how to develop a more balanced musculature around the foot, refer to our online workshop "The Flat Footed Elephant".

Lower hip of non-stance leg to affect hip abductors, piriformis, lateral head of gastrocnemius, biceps femoris and peroneals.

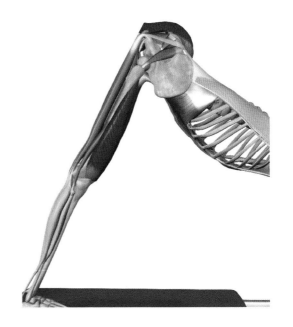

The Standing Calves 3.0

- **Standard:** Intermediate - Advanced • **Spring Tension:** Medium
- **Muscle Emphasis:** Entire calf group, hamstrings, gluteus maximus, adductor magnus

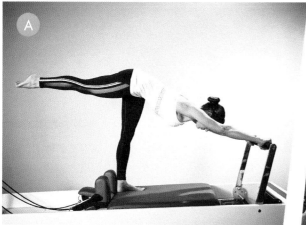

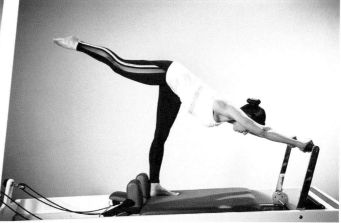

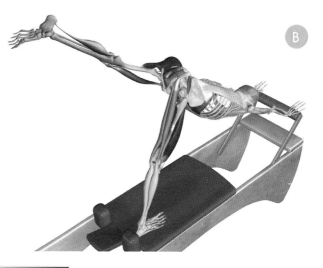

A & B. How to stretch

Press carriage away a little to POT as described in 2.0 on previous page, with both heels against shoulder rests. Lower chest then slowly, keeping hips level, begin to raise one leg to POT. Keep both legs straight

A & B. How to contract

Press the ball of the foot down into carriage.

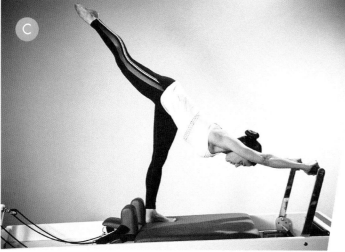

B & C. How to restretch

Slide carriage toward foot bar; i.e. more hip flexion. Lower chest. Lift rear leg further. Align leg, spine and arms.

What to watch out for:

- Arches of foot collapsing.
- Knee that is stretching/bending.
- Lifting/rotating hip of lifted leg – ensure hips stay level horizontally.

Gluteus maximus and adductor magnus work very strongly to lift and hold the leg in the air.

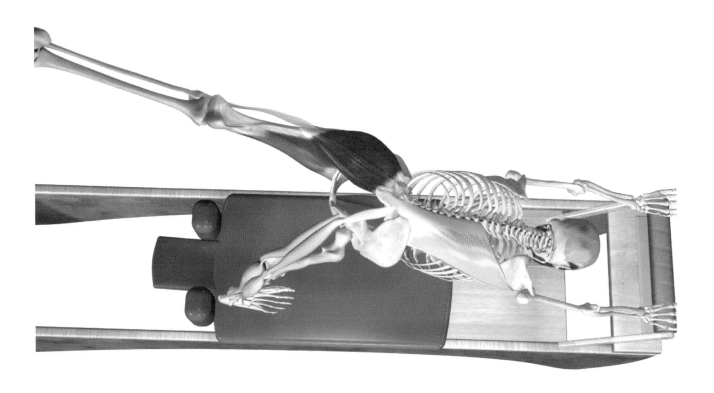

From the drone view, you can see down the posterior chain of the stretching leg from thoraco-lumbar fascia, sacrotuberous ligament, hamstrings, gastrocnemius and planter fascia.

Although certainly a stretch, a host of other muscles work strongly to maintain the position.

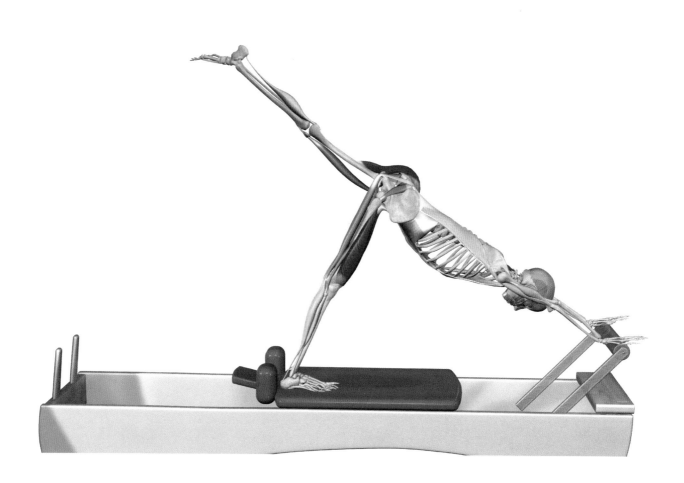

Notice the piriformis muscle stabilising the hip laterally, the triceps stabilising the shoulder and elbow joints, the gluteus maximus extending the hip, and the vastus lateralis supporting the knee joint.

On the front of the chest you can see pectoralis major and the rectus abdominus. The deepest abdominal muscle, transversus abdominus, along with the latissimus dorsi attatch to the thoracolumbar fascia in white.

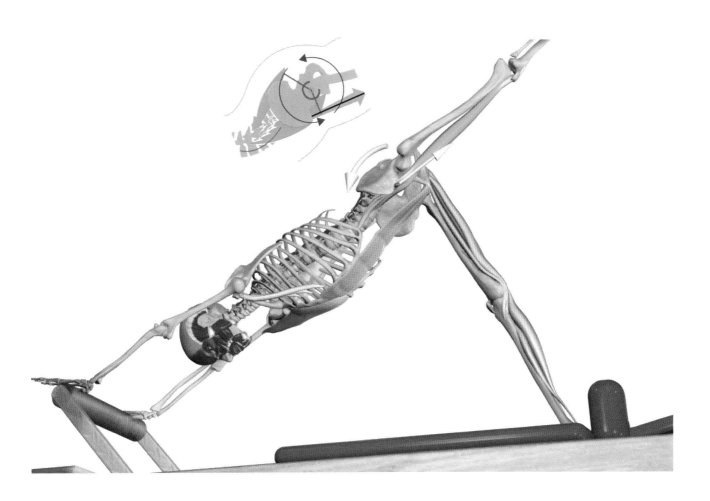

As the leg is lifted, the rectus femoris and illiopsoas are gradually stretched. Because of their attachment at the front of the pelvis, the pull is in an anterior direction (see arrows).

As a consequence, the stretch becomes stronger in the stance leg.

Variations

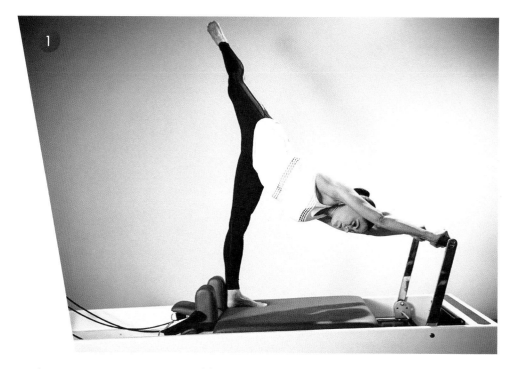

Try this creative variation. As you lift the leg and open the hips you may experience an adductor stretch (see Chapter 5). You may also feel some stretching around the abdominal region, especially if you exaggerate your breathing to expand the belly.

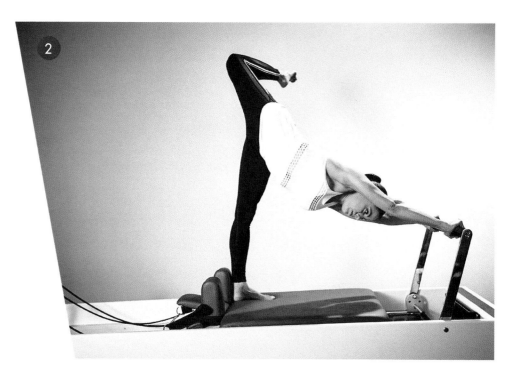

As you bend the lifted leg, you may feel stronger stretching sensations in the quadriceps and hip flexors of this leg (see Chapter 3).

The Standing Calves 4.0

- **Standard:** Advanced • **Spring Tension:** Medium
- **Muscle Emphasis:** Entire calf group, hamstrings, gluteus maximus, hip flexors and quadriceps of lifted leg

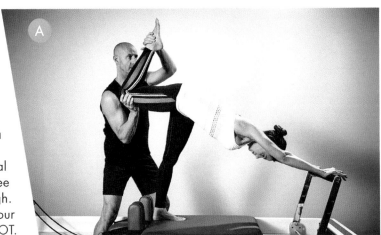

A. How to stretch

Take your leg into the final lifted position of version 3.0. Bend knee and have your partner lift the thigh. Have your partner take your foot toward your bottom at the same time to POT.

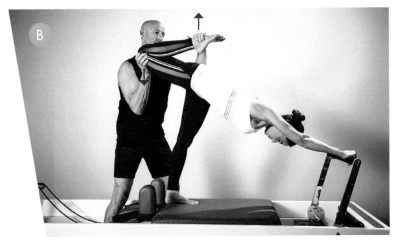

B. How to contract

Press thigh down into partner and foot up into partner.

C. How to restretch

Lift thigh and take foot further toward bottom.

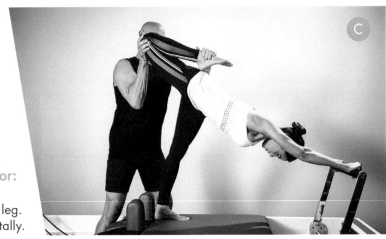

What to watch out for:

- Lifting/rotating hip of lifted leg. Ensure hips stay level horizontally.

As you bend the knee, the rectus femoris is gradually stretched. Because it attaches to the pelvis, it pulls the pelvis in an anterior direction.

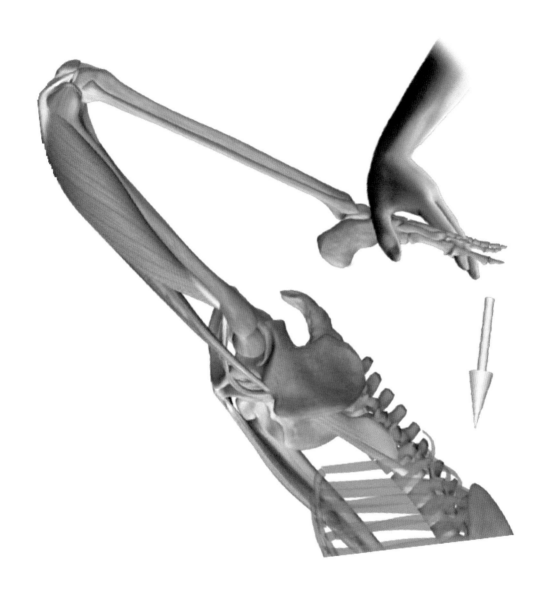

As a consequence, the stretch becomes stronger in the stance leg. In addition, the more the knee bends, the greater the stretch becomes in the quadriceps.

The Kneeling Calves

- Standard: Advanced • Spring Tension: Medium
- Muscle Emphasis: Entire calf group, hamstrings, gluteus maximus

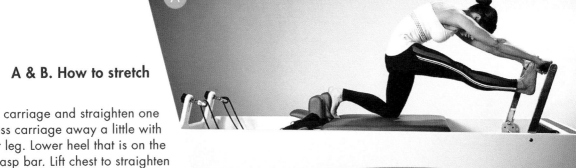

A & B. How to stretch

Kneel on carriage and straighten one leg. Press carriage away a little with the other leg. Lower heel that is on the bar. Clasp bar. Lift chest to straighten spine if possible.

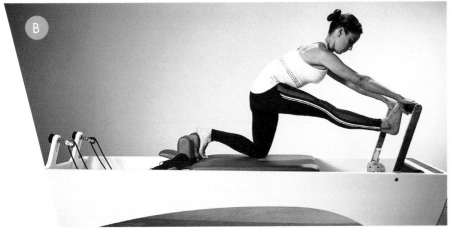

B. How to contract

Press thigh down into bar and ball of foot of front leg into bar.

B & C. How to restretch

Lift chest. Bend elbows to pull chest toward leg and lower heel further under bar if possible.

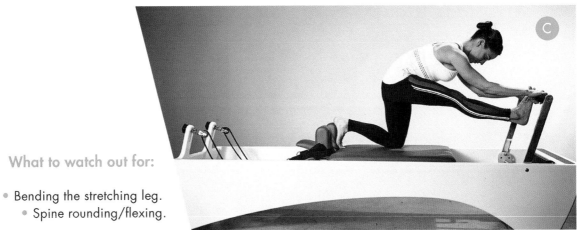

What to watch out for:

- Bending the stretching leg.
- Spine rounding/flexing.

The Lying Peroneals

- **Standard:** Any • **Spring Tension:** Light - Medium
- **Muscle Emphasis:** Peroneal muscle group

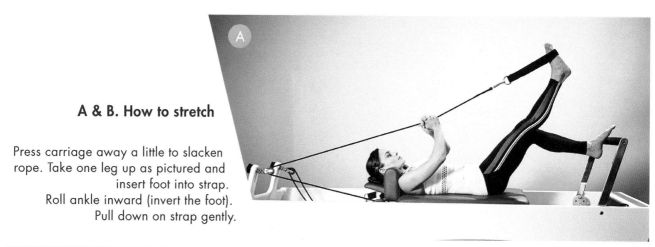

A & B. How to stretch

Press carriage away a little to slacken rope. Take one leg up as pictured and insert foot into strap.
Roll ankle inward (invert the foot).
Pull down on strap gently.

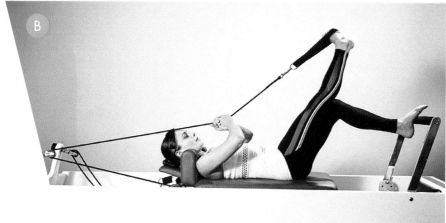

B. How to contract

Press foot back toward neutral position.

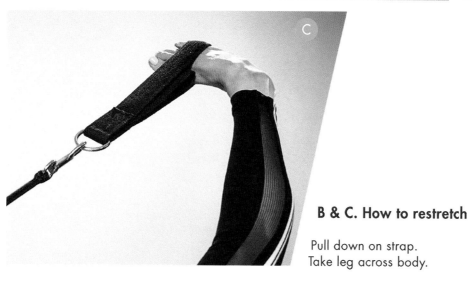

B & C. How to restretch

Pull down on strap.
Take leg across body.

The Standing Soleus

- Standard: Any
- Muscle Emphasis: Soleus, tibialis posterior

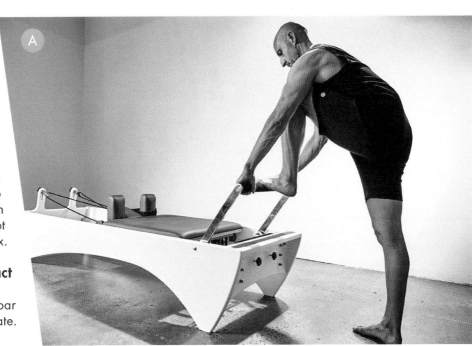

A. How to stretch

Place ball of one foot onto foot bar. Lower heel. Lean over thigh so that chest contacts thigh. Use arms to pull chest strongly onto thigh causing heel to lower and foot to dorsi flex.

A. How to contract

Press ball of foot into bar as if to accelerate.

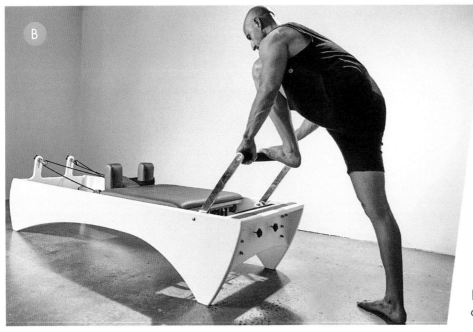

B. How to restretch

Bend elbows to pull chest onto leg with more force. Lower heel as much as possible.

Variation

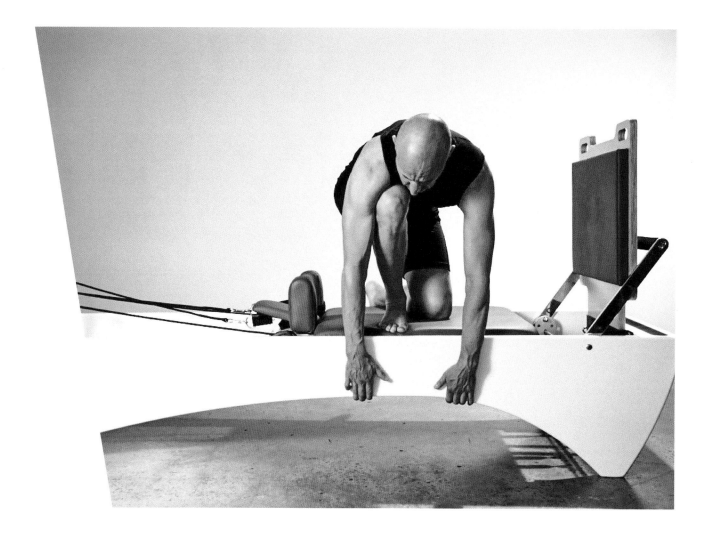

Kneeling version is the same except that the arms are pulling the chest by gripping under the carriage frame.

The Lying Peroneals 2.0

- **Standard:** Any • **Spring Tension:** Medium - Heavy
- **Muscle Emphasis:** Entire lateral/peroneal compartment

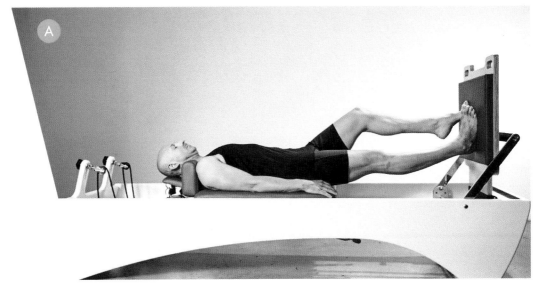

A. How to stretch

Press carriage away and place outside of one foot onto jump board. Bend other knee slowly, controlling carriage movement with this leg. As carriage slides in, allow foot to invert/ankle to "roll in".

A. How to contract: Try to turn foot back toward neutral position; i.e. evert the foot.

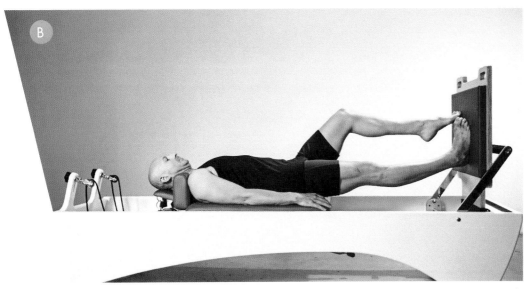

B. How to restretch

Allow support leg to bend further and carriage to travel in further.
Allow foot to invert further.

What to watch out for:

- Losing control of carriage movement. • Moving into stretch too quickly, "bouncing."

The Lying Tib Ant

- **Standard:** Any • **Spring Tension:** Medium - Heavy
- **Muscle Emphasis:** Entire anterior compartment including tibialis anterior, extensor hallucis and digitorum longus and brevis

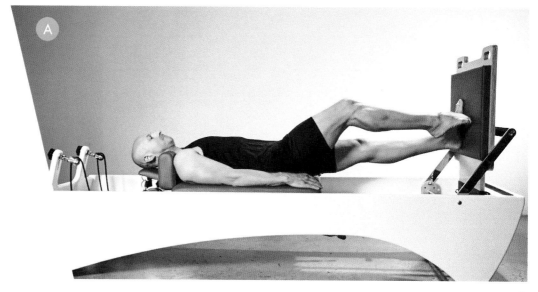

A. How to stretch

Press carriage away and place top of one foot onto Jump board. Bend other knee slowly, controlling carriage movement with this leg. As carriage slides in allow foot and toes to plantar flex.

A. How to contract: Press foot back into jump board toward neutral position i.e. dorsi flex the foot.

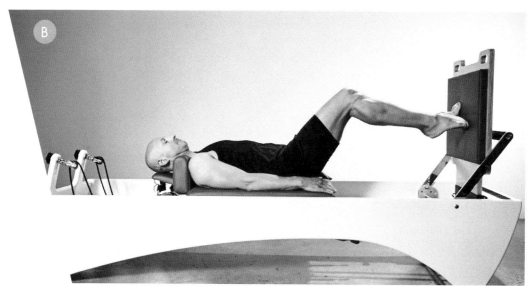

B. How to restretch

Allow leg to bend further and carriage to travel in further.
Allow foot to plantar flex further.

What to watch out for:

- Losing control of carriage movement. • Moving into stretch too quickly, "bouncing."

The Soleus

- **Standard:** Any • **Spring Tension:** Medium - Heavy
- **Muscle Emphasis:** Entire posterior compartment excluding gastrocnemius. Including tibialis posterior, flexor hallucis and digitorum longus.

How to stretch

Press carriage away and place foot onto jump board.
Bend knee slowly, controlling carriage movement with arms and leg.
As carriage slides in allow ankle/knee to bend further to POT.

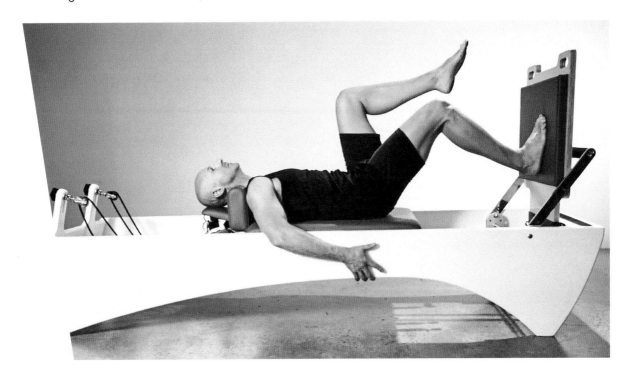

A. How to contract

Press foot into jump board;
i.e. plantar flex the foot.

B. How to restretch

Allow leg to bend further and carriage
to travel in further. Allow foot to dorsi
flex further. Use hands to pull carriage
in if additional stretch is required.

What to watch out for:

- Losing control of carriage movement.
- Moving into stretch too quickly, "bouncing".
- Arch collapsing to "flat footed" position.

Chapter Two

Hamstrings

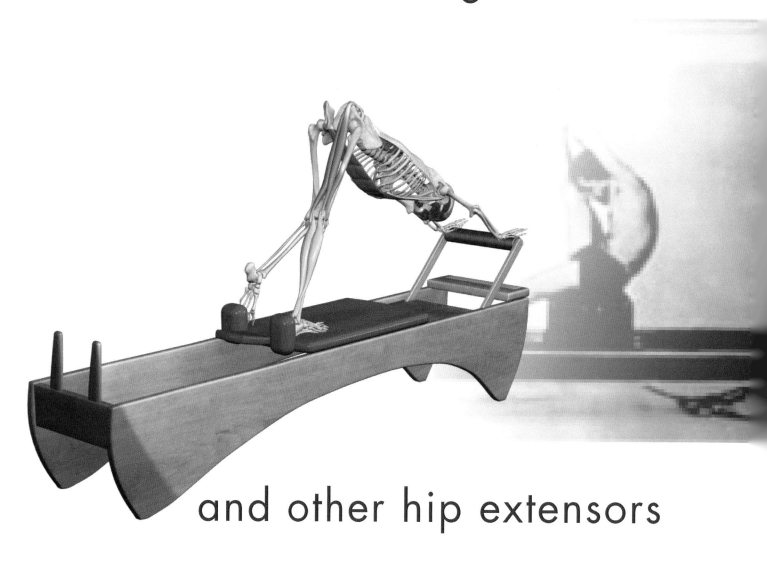

and other hip extensors

About this Chapter

There are many ways that I could have grouped the stretches in this chapter. I have chosen what makes sense anatomically and experientially. What is important is that you stretch all of the hamstring and hip extensor group. A program with variety will ensure that this is achieved.

The experience of stretching the hip extensors and knee flexors (Hamstrings, Gastrocnemius, Gluteus maximus, Adductor Magnus), with both a bent and straight leg approach, is qualitatively different. A look at the anatomical images will tell you why. Bent-limb stretches tend to focus their intensity in the Gluteus Maximus and Adductor Magnus muscles, rather than the Hamstrings. Straight leg stretches tend to focus more on the Hamstrings and Gastrocnemius, because, anatomically, they run across the knee joint. Both approaches need to be included in any flexibility training program. With this in mind, I have offered them in different groups, so that you are aware of which muscles you are targeting and are able to select from both groups in your practice.

In addition, there are across-the-body or "lateral" stretches, which are often variations on the previous two groups, but that have their own anatomical and experiential differences. "Lateral" stretches, where the leg is adducted or taken across the body, tend to move the locus of the stretch to the short and long head of the Biceps Femoris, muscles within the Hamstring group. In additio, you might also stretch the lateral head of Gastrocnemius, the Peroneals, and sometimes higher up in the hip into the Piriformis muscle. Again, they need to form part of any posterior leg flexibility training program.

Straight leg, bent leg and lateral stretches are divided into recommended standards. When devising a program, as mentioned above, I would strongly recommend at least one stretch from each group. You may also find that within one group you need to practise a beginner version, but within the next group you are able to practise a more advanced stretch. Don't be surprised by this: it is entirely normal because we are all asymmetrical, even within muscle groups.

If you continue to practise only one of the stretches, or only one of the groups, you may never discover this truth. Worse still, you may be perpetuating an already existing muscle imbalance.

Straight Leg Versions

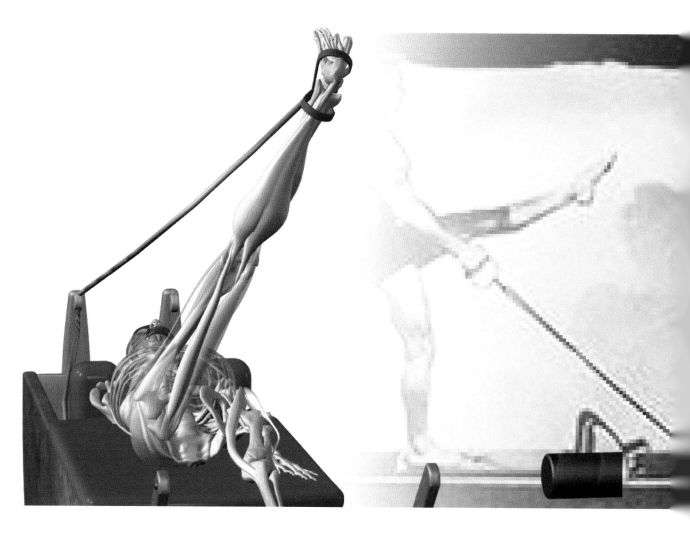

Straight Leg Versions / Lying HS

- **Standard:** Beginner & Intermediate • **Spring Tension:** Medium
- **Muscle Emphasis:** HS group, gastrocnemius, adductor magnus, horizontal leg-hip flexors

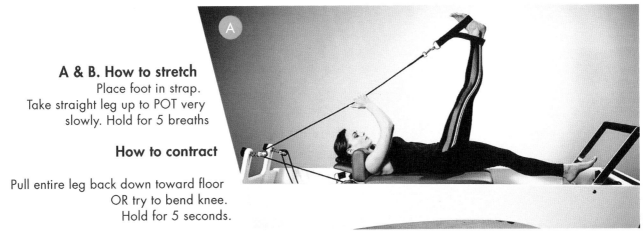

A & B. How to stretch
Place foot in strap.
Take straight leg up to POT very
slowly. Hold for 5 breaths

How to contract

Pull entire leg back down toward floor
OR try to bend knee.
Hold for 5 seconds.

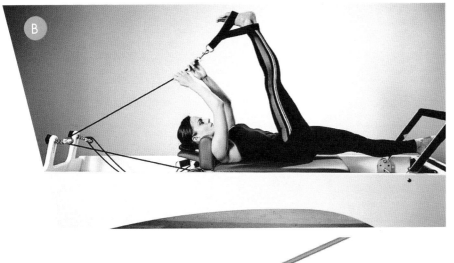

B. How to restretch

On a breath out, allow
carriage to slide in and hip to
flex further.

What to watch out for:

- Legs remain parallel.
- Hips remain square to leg/
neutral pelvis, no posterior or
lateral rotation.
- Legs remain straight.
- Bottom leg remains horizontal.

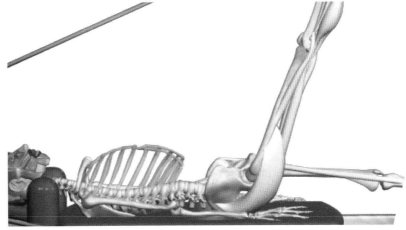

The posterior chain of leg muscles being stretched includes the Gastrocnemius, Hamstrings and extensor fibers of Gluteus Maximus.

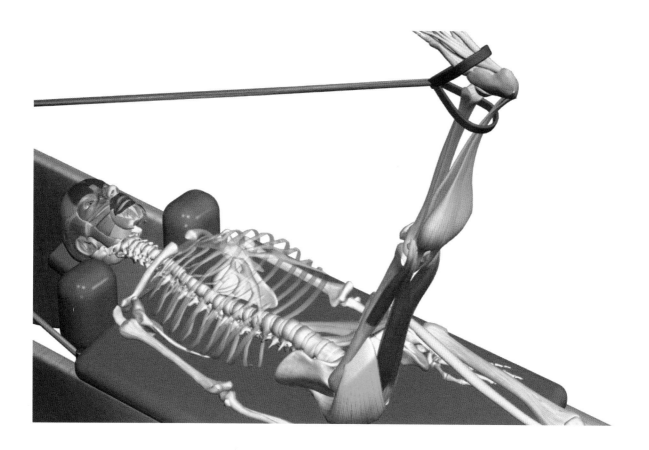

Keep an eye on the horizontal leg too. If it lifts, there could be stifness in sartorious, psoas and others.

The Standing Straight Leg Hamstrings

- **Standard:** Beginner - Intermediate • **Spring Tension:** Light - Medium
- **Muscle Emphasis:** Hamstrings, gastrocnemius, tibialis anterior, rear leg hip flexors

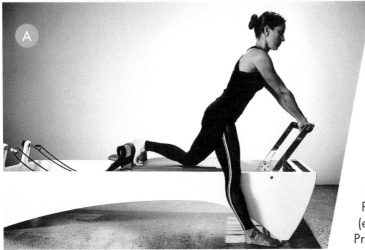

A. How to stretch

Keep legs in line with sit bones.
Press rear leg back to level hips; i.e. parallel (ensure two ASIS are level).
Press carriage away/lean hips back to POT.

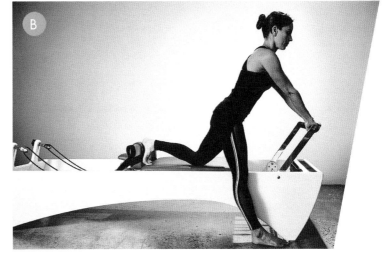

B. How to contract

Press front foot into floor.

C. How to restretch

Slide carriage further from resting position.

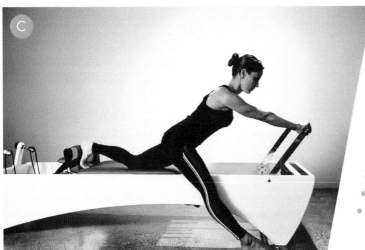

What to watch out for:

- Spine or low back flattening/rounding.
- Lateral pelvic rotation toward front leg.
- Front knee bending.
- Pelvis must remain neutral or anterior tilt.
- Hips to remain square to line of legs.

Variations

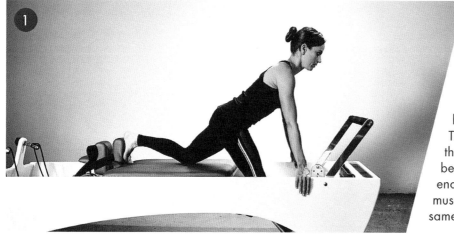

This sequence of photos shows an alternative position. The front leg is placed inside the carriage. The advantage of this position is that more of your body weight can be supported by your arms. This enables greater relaxation of the leg muscles under stretch. Instructions are same as above. **Try it!**

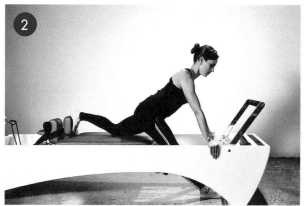

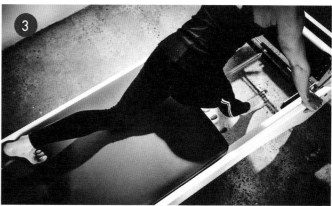

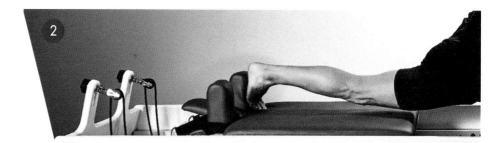

Variation Two

For greater intensity in both hamstrings and hip flexors, lift and straighten rear leg without lifting hips.

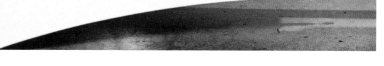

Reverse Straight Leg Hamstrings

- **Standard:** Intermediate & Advanced   • **Spring Tension:** Medium
- **Muscle Emphasis:** Gluteus maximus, hamstrings, muscles, tibialis anterior, hip flexors rear leg

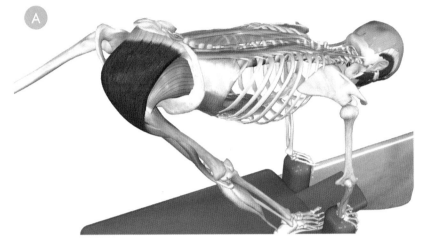

A. How to stretch

Place foot in front of shoulder rest.
Place rear leg onto foot bar.
Ensure legs parallel.
Press carriage away to POT.
Pelvis must remain neutral or anterior tilt.
Hips to remain square to line of legs.

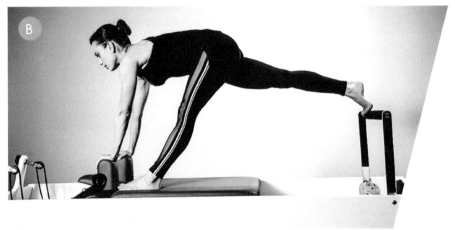

B. How to contract

Press front foot down into carriage.

C. How to restretch

Take carriage further from
resting position.
Keep pelvis in anterior tilt.

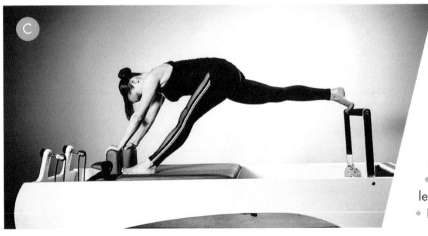

What to watch out for:

- Spine or low back flexing; i.e. rounding.
- Lateral pelvic rotation toward front leg; i.e. hips not square.
- Either knee bending.

Notice the posterior muscles of the thigh, from Gluteus Maximus, a portion of Medius to Hamstrings and calves. If you activate the Erector Spinae with the cue "lift your chest" or "point the sit bones up", the pelvis will be rotated forward/anterior, intensifying the stretch.

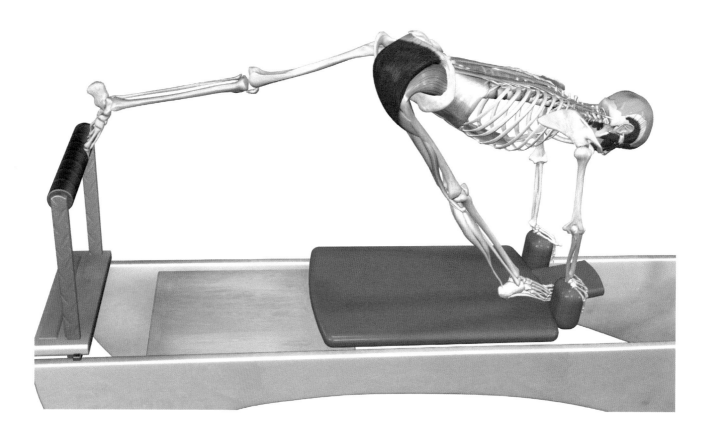

The transversus abdominus will stabilise the joints of the lower back if you gently "draw the navel toward the spine".

 To learn more about the transversus abdominus, take our online workshop titled "Safeguarding the Spine".

Laterals

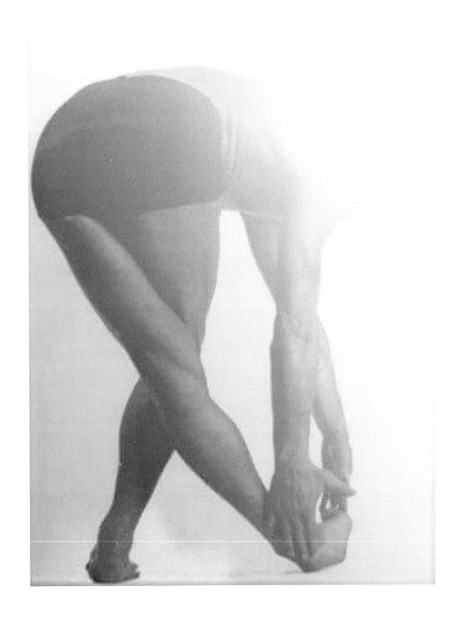

Lying Big Toe

- **Standard:** Beginner & Intermediate • **Spring Tension:** Medium
- **Muscle Emphasis:** Bicep femoris both heads, lateral gastrocnemius, external hip rotators, gluteus maximus, medius, minimus, horizontal leg-hip flexors

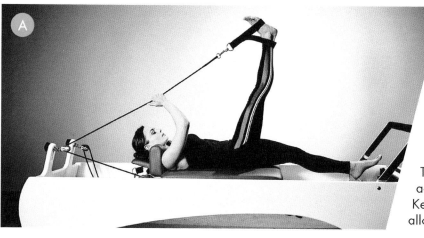

A & B. How to stretch

Take leg into flexion to POT, then slowly across midline of body.
Keep pelvis level horizontally (don't allow hip of lifted leg to lift).

B. How to contract

Press leg diagonally away from stretch position.

C. How to restretch

Take leg further into flexion, and further across midline of body.

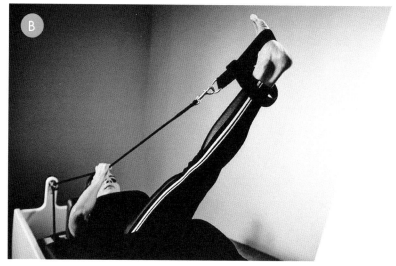

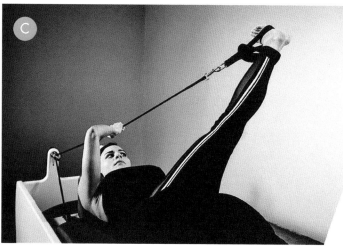

What to watch out for:

- Keep both hips on carriage.
- Keep pelvis neutral.
- Keep bottom leg horizontal.
- Keep stretching leg totally straight.
- Do not allow stretch leg to internally or externally rotate.

The posterior chain of muscles illustrated will stretch. The calves – in particular the lateral head of gastrocnemius, the lateral hamstrings including the short and **long head of** biceps femoris and even the pirifomis muscle of the hip – may feel a stretch.

The sartorius flexes, abducts and externally rotates the hip joint. If you find your lower leg tending toward any of these positions, stiffness in sartorius may be present.

Similarly, the tensor fascia lata flexes and abducts the thigh. If you show any signs of this motion, make note of it for later inspection.

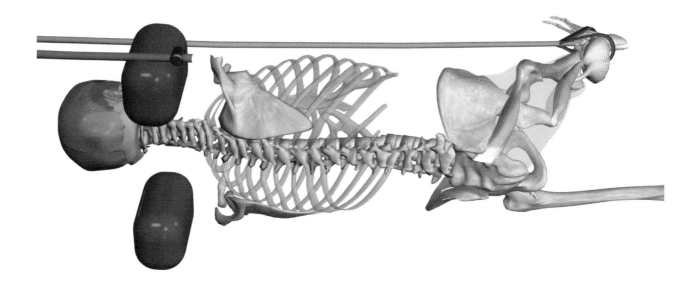

The "worm view" from under the reformer carriage illustrates the piriformis and long head of biceps femoris. You can see that by taking the leg across the body these two muscles will stretch.

Standing HS:
Straight Leg With Hip Shift

- **Standard:** Beginner & Intermediate ● **Spring Tension:** Light to Medium
- **Muscle Emphasis:** Lateral head of gastrocnemius, bicep femoris, external hip rotators, gluteus maximus, medius, minimus, rear leg hip flexors

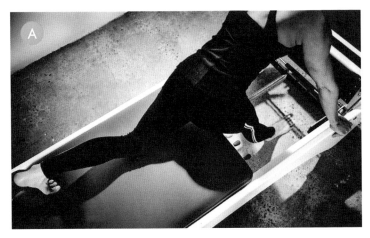

A & B. How to stretch

Start with leg on floor adducted;
i.e. toward midline of body.
Press carriage away to POT.
Pelvis must remain neutral or anterior tilt.
Shift hips laterally away from reformer.

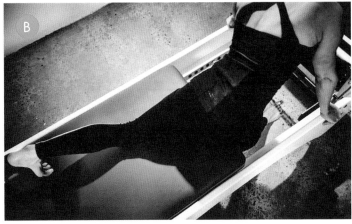

B. How to contract

Press front foot downward and away from reformer (extension & abduction).

C. How to restretch

Slide carriage further from resting position.
Shift hips further to side of reformer.

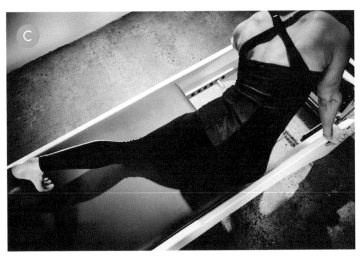

What to watch out for:

- Lateral rotation of pelvis instead of lateral shift.
- Low back flattening/flexing/rounding – posterior pelvic tilt.
- Front knee bending.

Reverse Big Toe

- **Standard:** Intermediate & Advanced • **Spring Tension:** Medium
- **Muscle Emphasis:** Lateral calves & hamstrings, external hip rotators, gluteals, tibialis anterior hip flexors rear leg

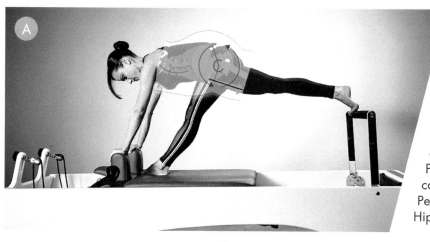

A & B. How to stretch

Place foot on carriage in line with foot on foot bar; i.e. adducted across center of body.
Press carriage away with leg on carriage to POT.
Pelvis must remain neutral or anterior tilt.
Hips must remain square to line of rear leg.

B. How to contract

Press foot on reformer down and rearward.

How to restretch (not shown)

Take carriage further from resting position.
Keep pelvis in anterior tilt.

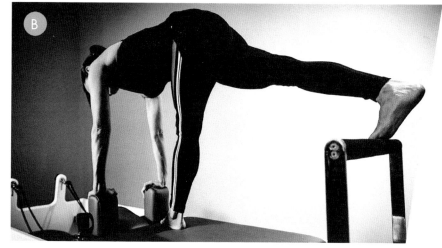

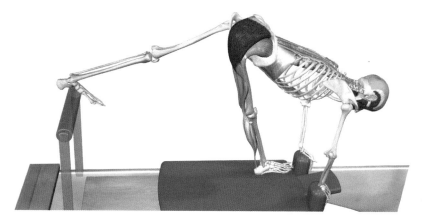

What to watch out for:

- Lateral rotation of pelvis toward leg on carriage.
- Spine flattening/flexing/rounding –posterior pelvic tilt.
- Front knee bending.
- Foot inverting.

Bent Leg
Hamstrings

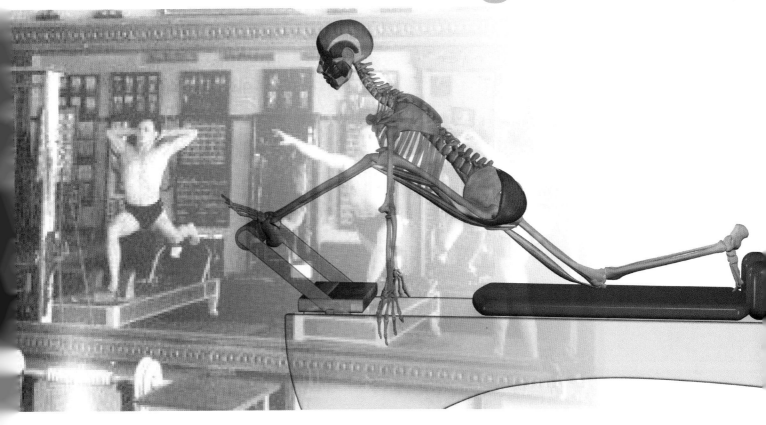

Standing HS Bent Leg

- **Standard:** Beginner & Intermediate ● **Spring Tension:** Light to Medium
- **Muscle Emphasis:** HS group, gluteus maximus-extensor fibers, adductor magnus, rear leg hip flexors

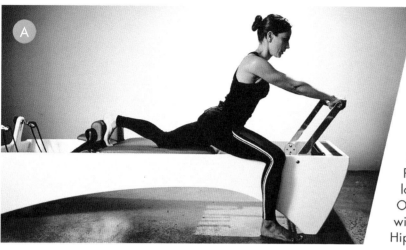

A & B. How to stretch

Place foot on floor toward front of reformer. Press carriage away with rear leg and lower hips maximally with front knee bent. Once in position, try to straighten front leg without lifting hips to POT.
Hips must remain square to line of rear leg.

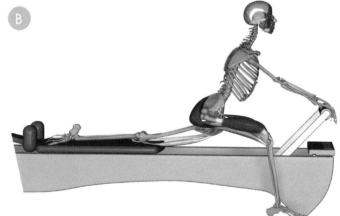

B. How to contract
Press both feet down.

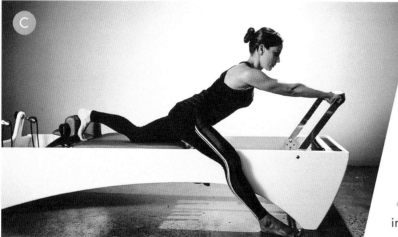

C. How to restretch

Slide carriage further out by trying to straighten front leg. Place hands either on bar or side of reformer.

What to watch out for:

- Hips lifting.
- Not lowering hips maximally in initial position.

Use This Link to See Video: https://www.youtube.com/watch?v=-mlVVwA4vlc

Variations

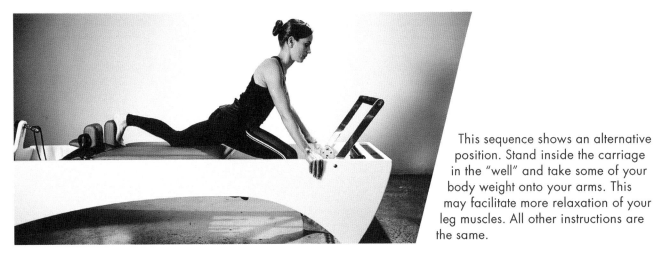

This sequence shows an alternative position. Stand inside the carriage in the "well" and take some of your body weight onto your arms. This may facilitate more relaxation of your leg muscles. All other instructions are the same.

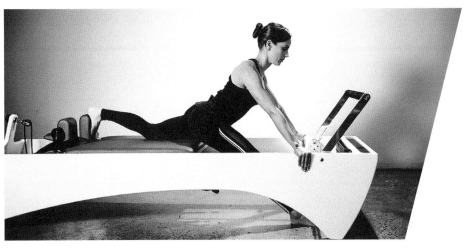

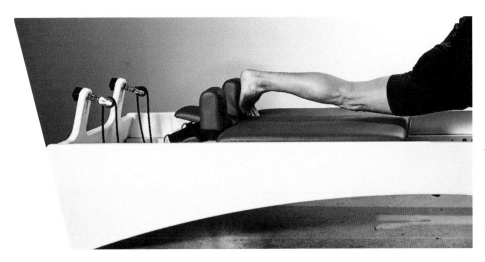

Variation Two

To intensify, tighten quadriceps of rear leg and lift knee cap without lifting thigh from carriage.

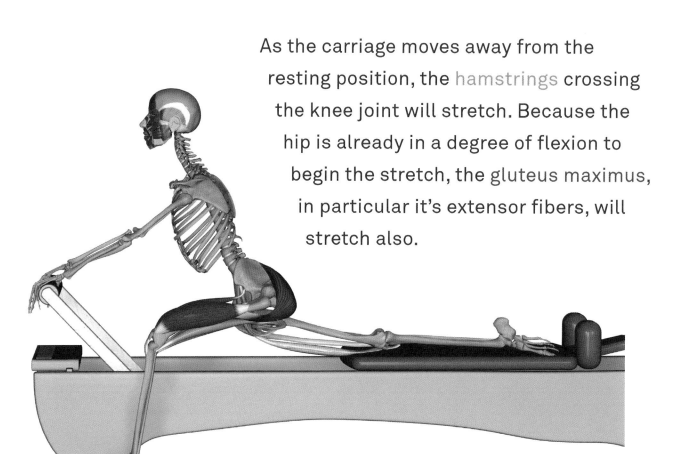

As the carriage moves away from the resting position, the hamstrings crossing the knee joint will stretch. Because the hip is already in a degree of flexion to begin the stretch, the gluteus maximus, in particular it's extensor fibers, will stretch also.

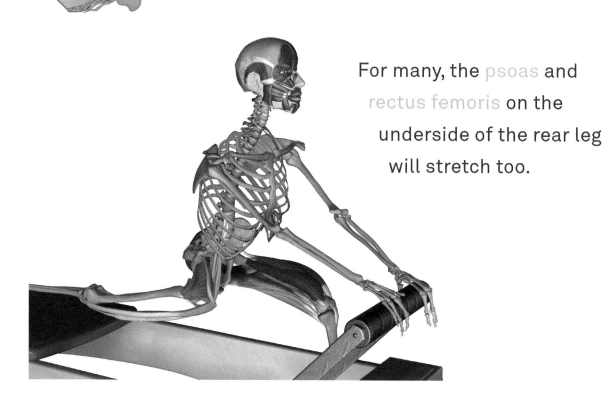

For many, the psoas and rectus femoris on the underside of the rear leg will stretch too.

Kneeling Bent Leg Hamstring

- **Standard:** Intermediate & Advanced • **Spring Tension:** Medium
- **Muscle Emphasis:** HS group, gluteus maximus, adductor magnus, rear leg hip flexors

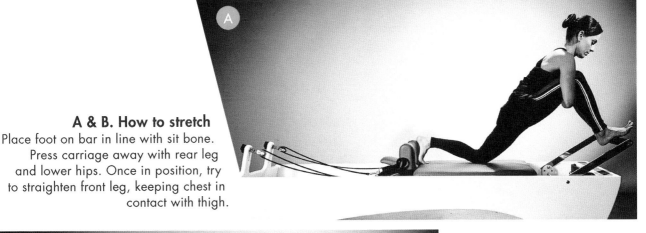

A & B. How to stretch
Place foot on bar in line with sit bone. Press carriage away with rear leg and lower hips. Once in position, try to straighten front leg, keeping chest in contact with thigh.

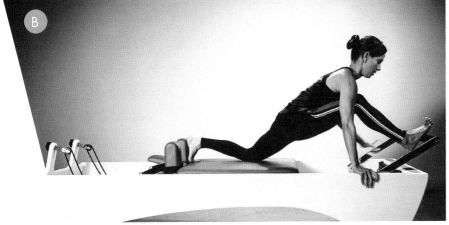

B. How to contract

Press both feet down.

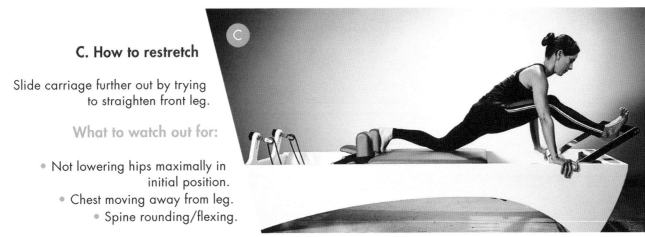

C. How to restretch

Slide carriage further out by trying to straighten front leg.

What to watch out for:

- Not lowering hips maximally in initial position.
- Chest moving away from leg.
- Spine rounding/flexing.

Variation

This photograph shows an advanced variation. Lift the rear knee, without lifting the hips, for a stronger stretch in all muscles groups involved.

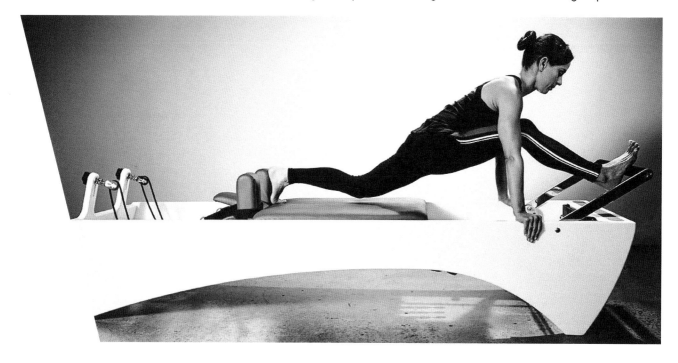

As the rear knee lifts, tension generated in the rectus femoris rotates the pelvis forward/anteriorly, increasing the stretch in the hamstrings and glutues maximus.

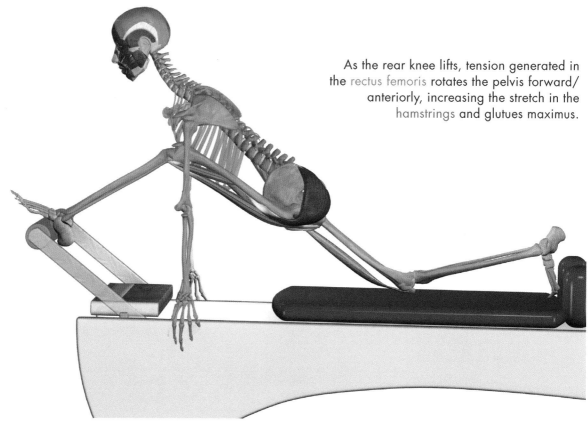

The Russian

- **Standard:** Intermediate & Advanced • **Spring Tension:** Medium
- **Muscle Emphasis:** Hamstrings, gluteus maximus extensor fibers, adductor magnus, hip flexors rear leg

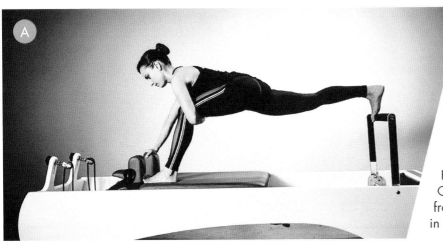

A. How to stretch

Place foot on in front of shoulder rest in line with sit bone. Press carriage away with rear leg and lower hips. Place chest on thigh. Keep legs parallel.
Once in position, try to straighten front leg on carriage, keeping chest in contact with thigh.

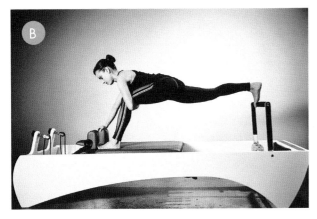

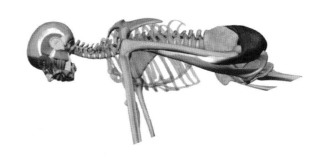

B. How to contract Press front foot down and backward as if to flex knee further.

C. How to restretch

Slide carriage further out by tying to straighten front leg.

What to watch out for:

- Not lowering hips maximally in initial position.
- Chest moving away from leg.
- Back leg bending.
- Spine flexing/bending.
- Pelvis rotating laterally toward front foot.

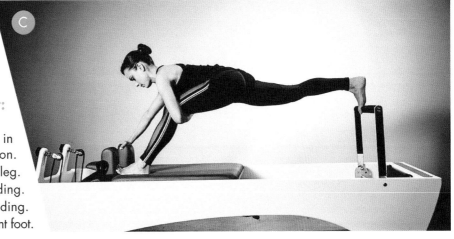

Chapter Three

Hip Flexors & Quadriceps

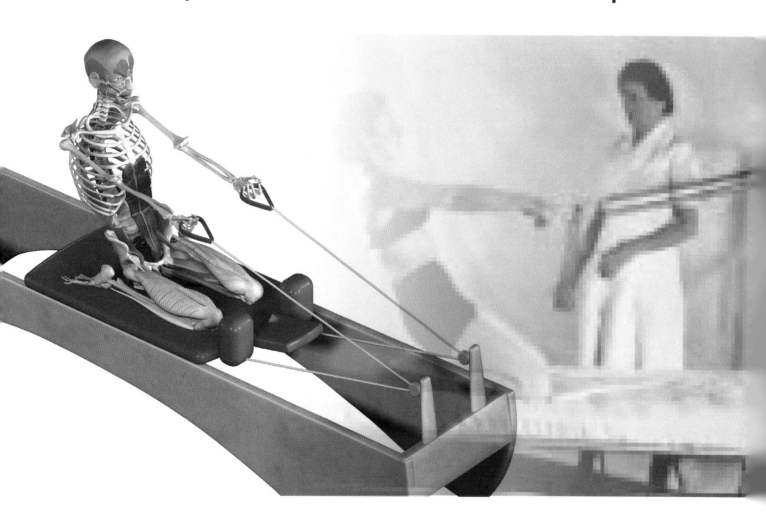

About this Chapter

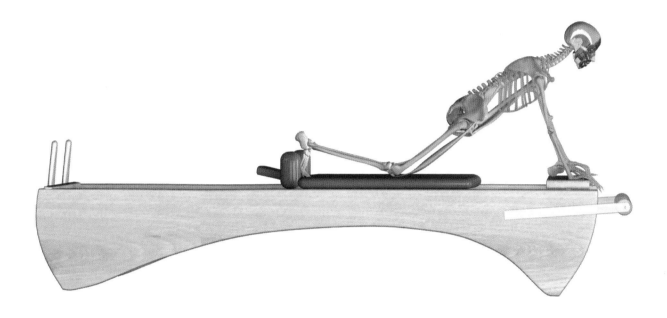

There are 11 muscles that can act to flex the hip joint. All of them pull at slightly different angles on the leg bone or femur. As a consequence, you need to stretch the thigh and pelvis at different angles. Many of the stretches in this chapter have variations for this reason.

Experiment with them all to start with. You may find, as you did with the hamstrings, that some stretches and variations yield strong sensations while others feel "nah, not much". That is entirely normal. Your body is its past; a precise representation of how you have used it. As a consequence, it will never be entirely symmetrical.

Part B of this chapter includes the Quadriceps. Remember that only the Rectus Femoris crosses the hip joint, so only it will be stretched in part A, where the hip joint is in extension without much knee flexion. In part B, when the knee is flexed as well, the other quadriceps will stretch also.

The hip flexors and Rectus Femoris exert a strong anterior pull on the pelvis affecting its placement, with repercussions through the entire spinal column. For more detail on this, refer to "Innovations in Pilates, Therapeutic Muscle stretching on the Pilates Reformer", and the online workshops on our website.

Part A
Hip Flexors Without Quadriceps

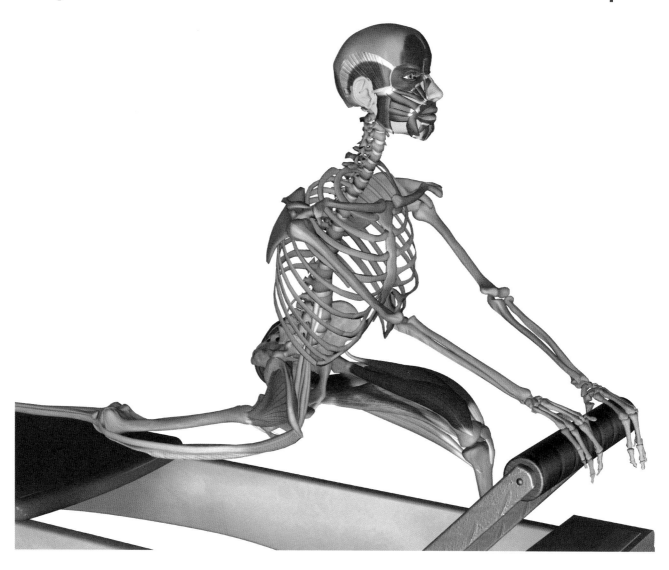

The Standing Lunge

- **Standard:** Beginner • **Spring Tension:** Light-Medium
- **Muscle Emphasis:** Illiopsoas, rectus femoris, secondary-underside of front leg-hamstrings, gluteus maximus, adductor magnus

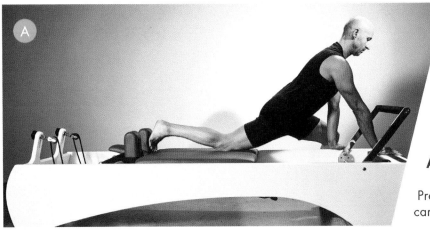

A. How to stretch

Press carriage away, bend front knee and lower hips maximally. Use arms to support body weight. Ensure hips stay square to line of legs.

A. How to contract

Press back foot and knee down into carriage, and front foot.

B & C. How to restretch

Lower hips further.
Tilt pelvis toward posterior tilt.
Lift rear knee without lifting hips
(Photo C).
Contract abdominals.

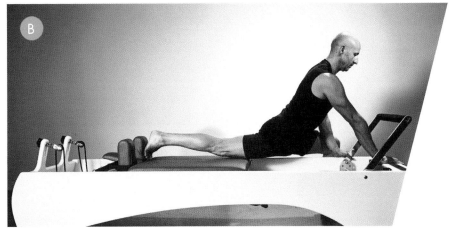

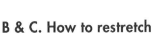

What to watch out for:

- Low back extension.
- Hips not lowering in beginning position.
- Angle at front knee too narrow – keep foot in front of knee, not underneath it, lifting hips along with lifting rear knee.

Variation One & Two

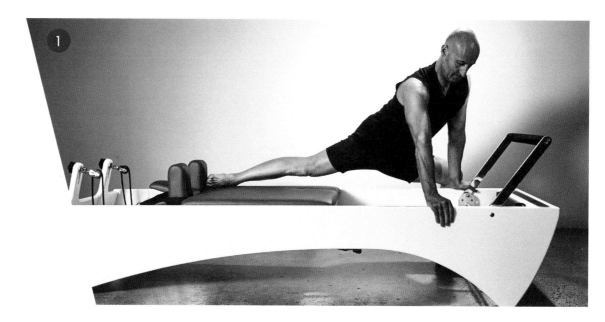

Variation One

Open hips to expose the inside of the rear leg, the entire adductor group. Explore slowly.

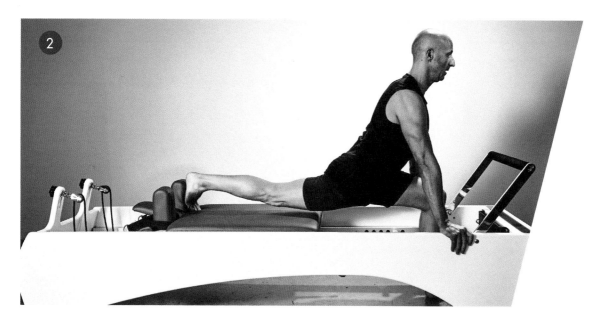

Variation Two

Follow the instructions above, but stand inside the reformer as pictured. You may find that this version allows the arms to support you better. The more of your body weight you can support with your arms, the more that your hip muscles will be able to relax.

Variation Three

"Over-rotate" the pelvis to shift the stretch to the outside of the pelvic girdle. The focus will now be on the tensor fascia lata and anterior portions of gluteus medius and minimus.

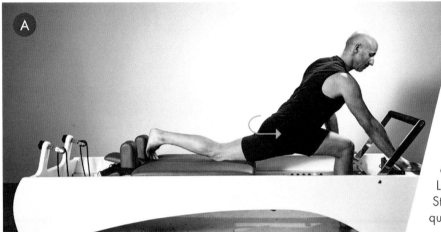

A & B. How to stretch

Follow the same set-up as above, but change the initial foot position.
Stand inside the reformer and place the right rear foot on the left shoulder rest. The legs will be in the same line, rather than parallel as in the above stretch.
Lower hips maximally.
Straighten rear leg by contracting quads (Photo B).

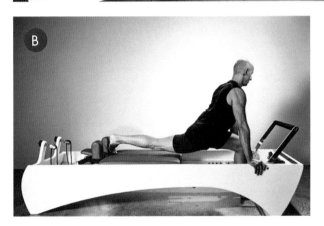

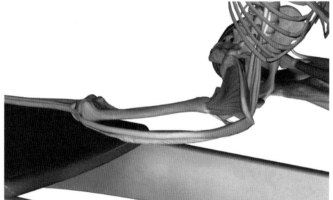

C. How to stretch

Rotate the right side of the pelvis and trunk toward the foot bar as much as you can.
Contract the abdominals by drawing the navel toward the spine.
Tuck the tail bone under.

Once you find the stretch, hold for 90 seconds. Explore subtle shifts too.

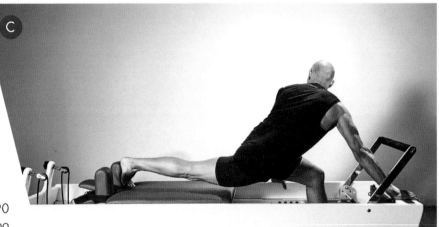

The Lunge 2.0

- **Standard:** Intermediate & Advanced • **Spring Tension:** Light - Medium
- **Muscle Emphasis:** - Illiopsoas, rectus femoris, secondary- underside of front leg-hamstrings, gluteus maximus, adductor magnus

A. How to stretch

Press carriage away, bend front knee
to just over 90 degrees.
Lower hips maximally.
Press back leg away while maintaining
angle at front leg.
Arms inside front leg.
Lift chest to engage lats.

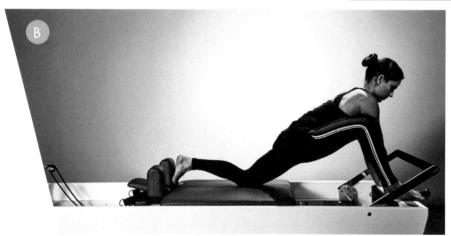

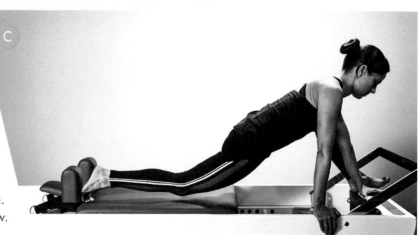

B. How to contract

Press back foot and knee
down into carriage.
Press front foot into reformer.

C. How to restretch

Lower hips further. Lift rear knee
without lifting hips. Move hands for
more support if required.

What to watch out for:

- Low back extension.
- Hips not lowering in beginning position.
- Angle at front knee too narrow.

The Lunge 2.0 is a strong stretch for the rectus femoris and adductor magnus seen below.

Psoas major can also be seen.

Keeping the back straight by lifting the chest will engage the latissimus dorsi. This will tension the thoraco-lumbar fascia and support the lower back region.

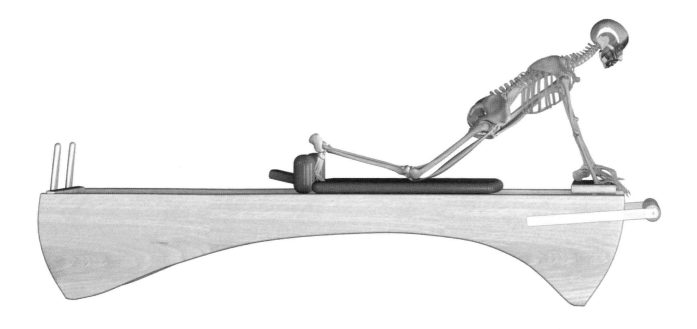

▶ See Chapter One for Thoraco-Lumbar fascia images.

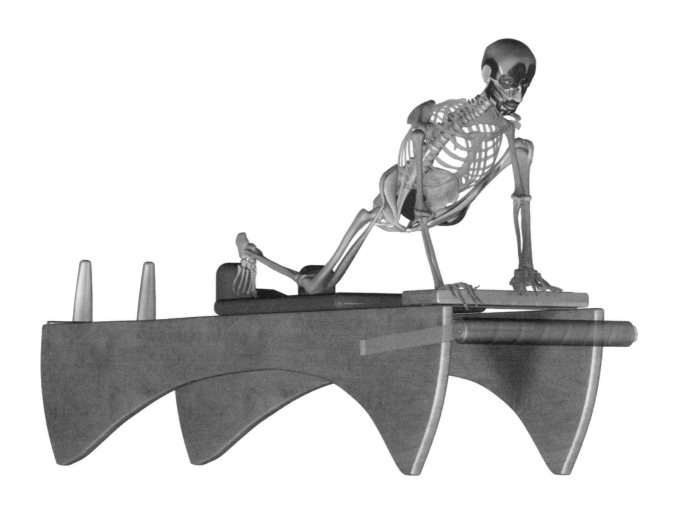

Rectus femoris attaches from two points just under the front tip of the pelvis known as the ASIS.

The psoas major can be seen attaching to the front of the lumbar vertebra. It joins with the illiacus and then wraps around to insert onto the lessor trochantor of the femur.

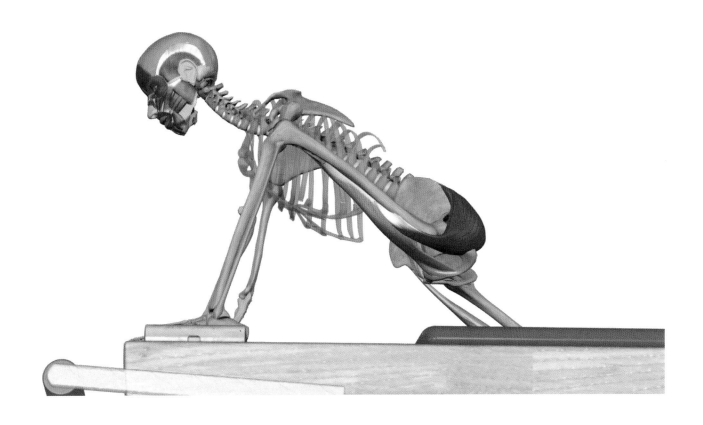

A portion of gluteus maximus inserts onto the leg bone or femur. As a result, when the leg is strongly flexed like this it will stretch.

The adductor magnus once crossed the knee joint. Over time, its tendon became the lateral knee ligament. A portion of it will also stretch in this position.

Hip Flexors, "The Classic"!

- **Standard:** Intermediate to Advanced • **Spring Tension:** Light - Medium
- **Muscle Emphasis:** Illiopsoas, rectus femoris, adductor longus, pectineus,
  Secondary- underside of front leg-hamstrings, gluteus maximus, adductor magnus

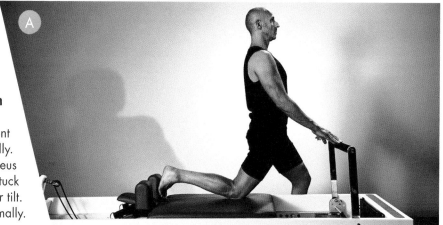

A. How to stretch

Press carriage away and ensure front
hip bones are level horizontally.
Tighten abdominal (ASIS) and gluteus
maximus muscles and tuck
tail under to achieve posterior tilt.
Once achieved, lower hips maximally.

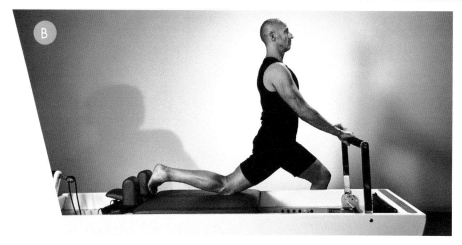

A & B. How to contract

Press back foot and knee down
into carriage.

B. How to restretch

Lower hips further. Press arms
down into foot bar to engage
abdominals.

What to watch out for:

- Low back extension
- Loss of posterior tilt.
- Thoracic flexion.

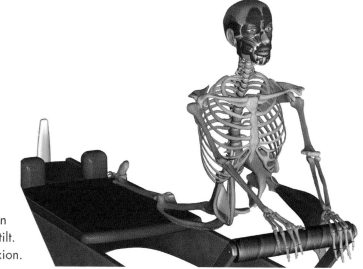

The primary hip flexor is illiopsoas. As you tilt the pelvis posteriorly, its origins on the lumbar spine and inside the pelvis move away from its insertions on the femur, helping to create the stretch.

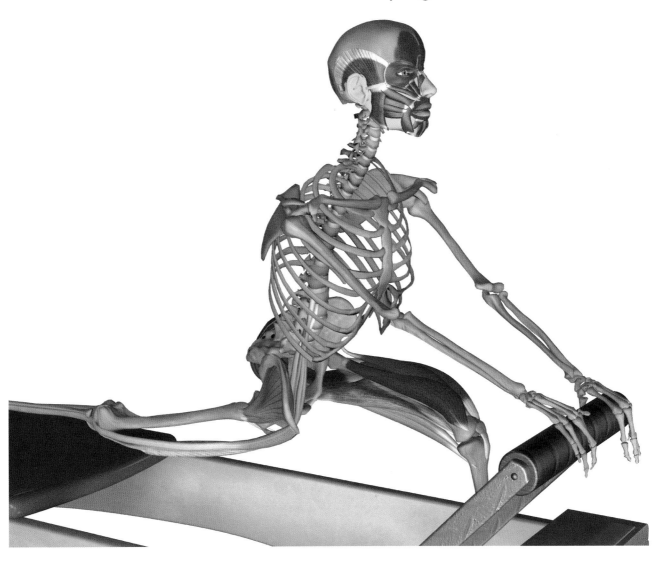

The quadriceps muscles will move the carriage away. By contracting them, the muscles on the underside of the front leg, hamstrings and addcutor magnus, will be inhibited via a process called reciprocal inhibition. This enables them to stretch more deeply.

This image shows the outside/lateral hip flexors: gluteus medius, gluteus minimus and tensor fascia lata. The anterior fibres of the abductors – medius and minimus – are synergists for hip flexion.

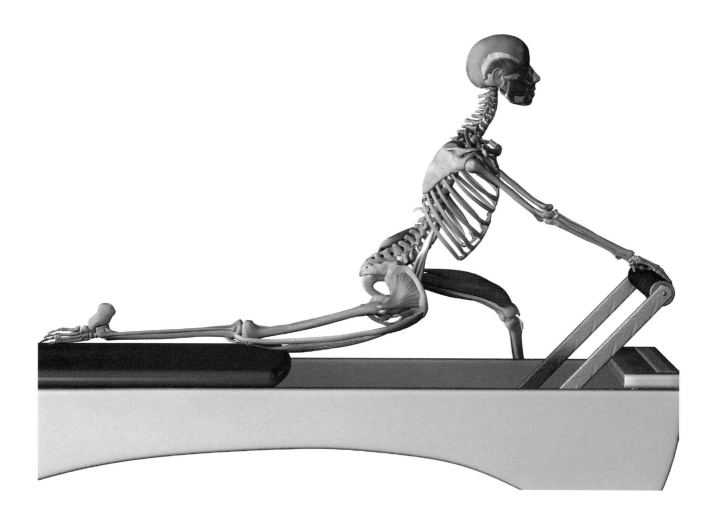

You can also see rectus femoris.

Variations

Rotate hip that is stretching toward foot bar to stretch tensor fascia lata and anterior fibres of gluteus minimus and medius.

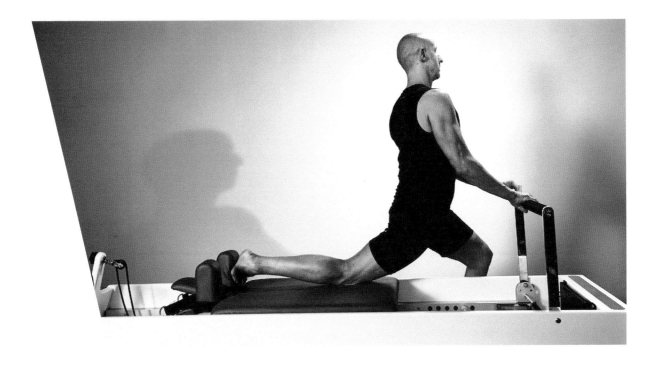

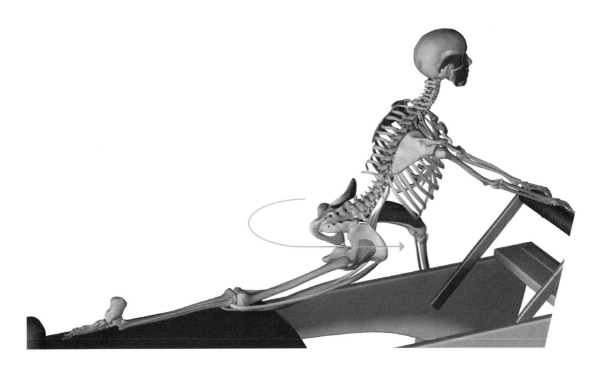

Hip Flexor Advanced

- **Standard:** Advanced • **Spring Tension:** Medium
- **Muscle Emphasis:** All hip flexors and abdominal muscles on same side, glutues maximus, hamstrings and adductor magnus of front leg

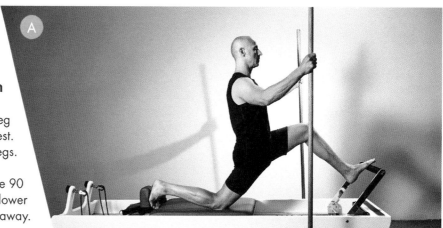

A. How to stretch

Place front foot on bar and rear leg against shoulder rest. Lift chest. Square hips to line of legs.

Move carriage away to achieve 90 degree angle at front knee and lower hips maximally. Press back leg away.

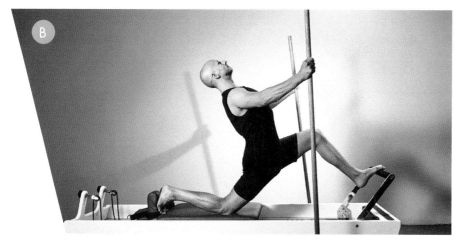

A. How to contract

Press front foot down into bar. Press rear knee and foot down into carriage.

B. How to restretch

Maintain 90 degree joint angle at front leg. Press rear leg away and lower hips as much as possible. Lift chest and lean backwards. Take deep abdominal breaths to expand abdominal cavity.

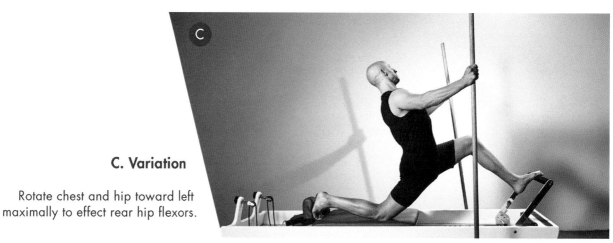

C. Variation

Rotate chest and hip toward left maximally to effect rear hip flexors.

Part B

Hip Flexors & Quadriceps

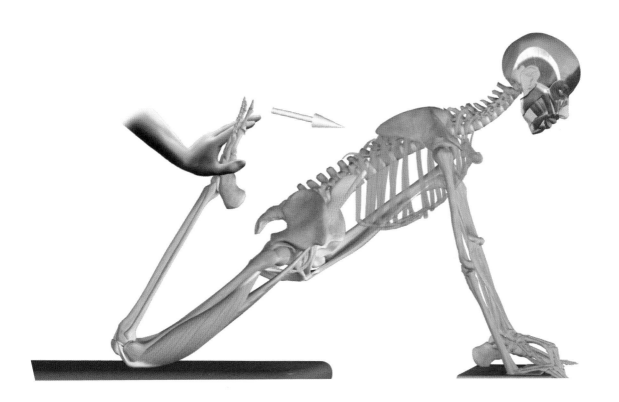

The Lunge 3.0 with Rec Fem & Quads

- **Standard:** Intermediate to Advanced • **Spring Tension:** Light - Medium
- **Muscle Emphasis:** Illiopsoas, rectus femoris, quadriceps, secondary- underside of front leg-hamstrings, gluteus maximus, adductor magnus

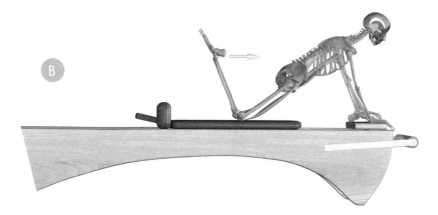

A. How to stretch

Press carriage away, bend front knee to just over 90 degrees. Lower hips maximally. Press back leg away while maintaining angle at front leg.

Place hands inside front leg. Lift back foot slowly toward bottom. Partner to press on pelvis to keep hips low.

B. How to contract

Press back foot away from bottom. Press back knee down into carriage. Press front foot into reformer.

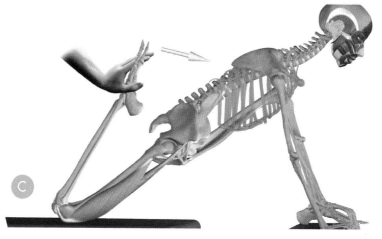

C. How to restretch

Lower hips further. Take rear foot toward bottom.

What to watch out for:

- Hips not lowering in beginning position.
  - Angle at front knee too narrow.
    - Leaning hips backward.

Thigh Stretch

- **Standard**: Any • **Spring Tension**: Heavy
- **Muscle Emphasis**: Rectus femoris, quadriceps, tibialis anterior, toe extensors

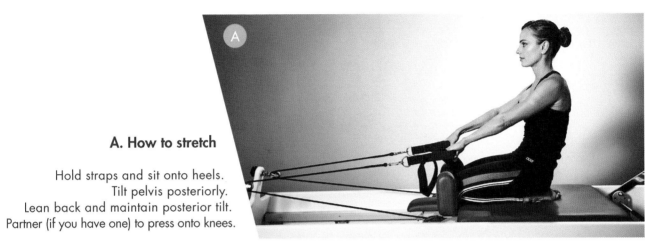

A. How to stretch

Hold straps and sit onto heels.
Tilt pelvis posteriorly.
Lean back and maintain posterior tilt.
Partner (if you have one) to press onto knees.

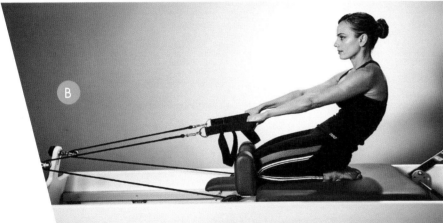

B. How to contract

Press back feet and toes into
carriage. Press shins down
into carriage.

C. How to restretch

Maintain pelvic tilt
and lean further back.
Contract abdominal muscles

What to watch out for:

- Low back extension.
- Legs moving apart (abducting).
- Knees lifting.

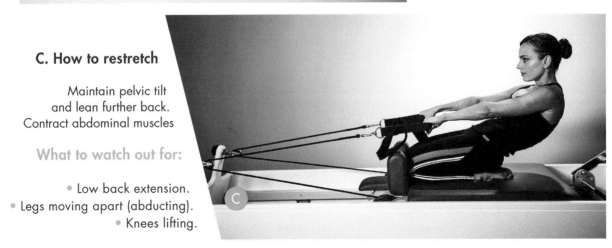

The rectus abdominus tilts the pelvis backwards/ posteriorly if contracted. Because the rectus femoris attaches to the pelvis, this action will deepen the stretch in this muscle.

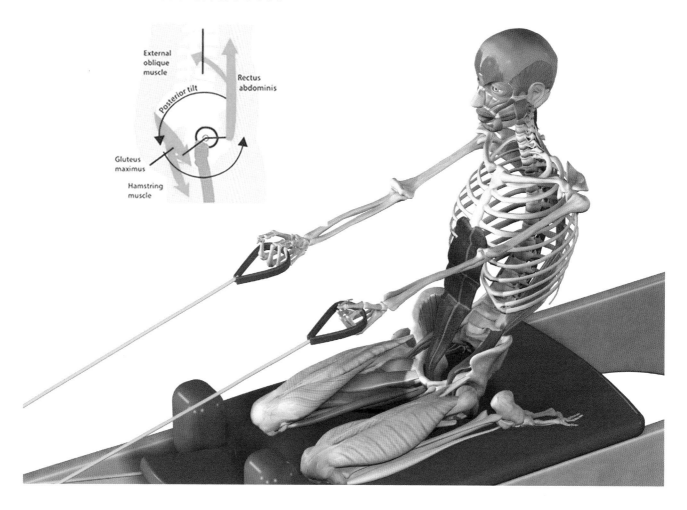

The erector spinae may also feel a stretch because the spine is strongly flexed. Note the large size of the quadriceps muscles, the adductor muscles and the illiacus originating inside the pelvic bowl.

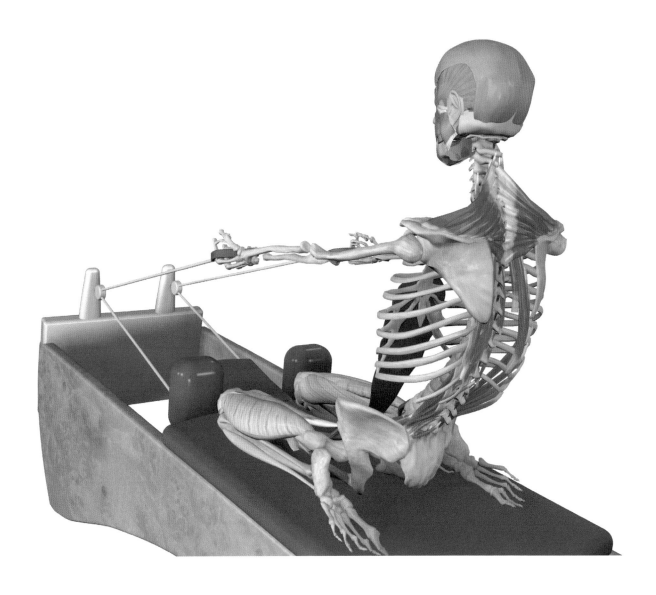

As you lean further back (if your quadriceps muscles allow it), your shoulder blades will move apart. This is called protraction or abduction.

The upper and middle trapezius muscles will stretch when this occurs.

Godzilla

- **Standard:** Intermediate to Advanced • **Spring Tension:** Light - Medium
- **Muscle Emphasis:** Rectus femoris, quadriceps, tibialis anterior, toe extensors

A. How to stretch

Hold rear foot and place shin against shoulder rest. Tilt pelvis posteriorly. Square hips to line of leg. Pull rear foot toward bottom.

A. How to contract

Press back foot and toes into hand. Press rear knee down into carriage.

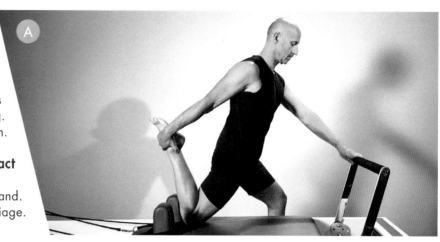

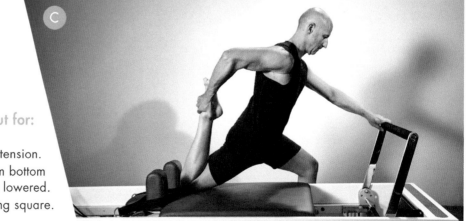

B & C. How to restretch

Maintain pelvic tilt and pull foot toward bottom. Lower hips by bending front leg.

What to watch out for:

- Low back extension.
- Foot moving away from bottom as hips are lowered.
- Hips remaining square.

Chapter Four

Gluteals

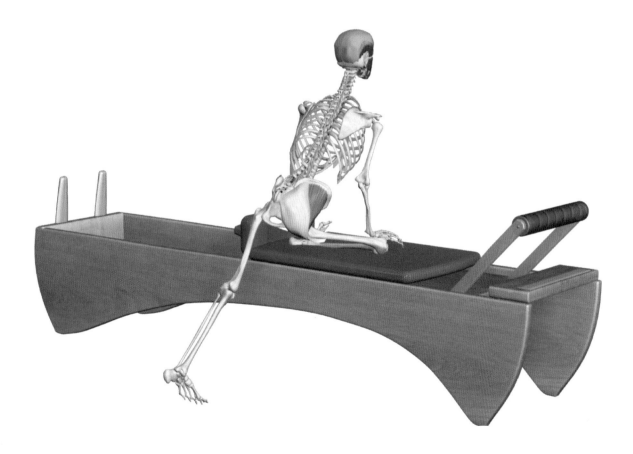

About the Gluteals

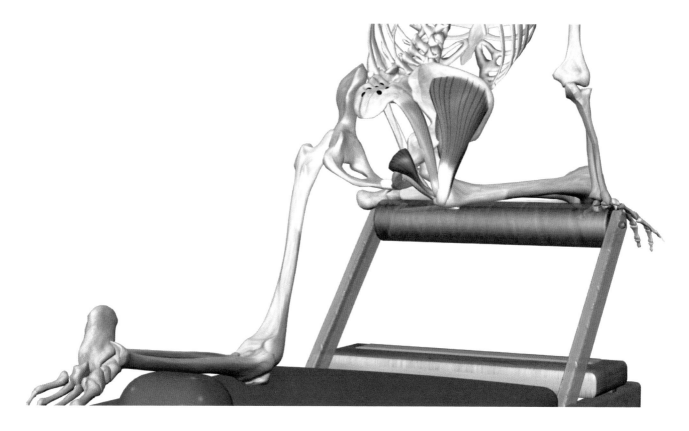

"Gluteals" is a rather nebulous term to describe the large number of muscles in this region. Included are the gluteus maximus medius and minimus and the six "short external rotators" that also provide stability to the posterior side of the hip joint. This group includes the piriformis, obturator internus and externus, gemellus superior and inferior, and quadratus femoris.

All of these muscles have primary roles in the so-called anatomical position, but their actions can change considerably when motion is performed outside of the anatomical position. This is because

their line of force changes. As with the other muscle groups studied so far, you need to explore a variety of hip and femoral joint angles. This will shift the locus of the stretch around the region and ensure, as much as possible, that each of the muscles in the group is at some point the "prime target".

This is the essence of stretching work, to locate your tight regions, muscles, and fibres within muscles. This essence cannot be achieved without directing your attention inward and exploring.

The Lying Gluteals

- **Standard:** Beginner • **Spring Tension:** Medium
- **Muscle Emphasis:** Gluteal group including deep hip rotators

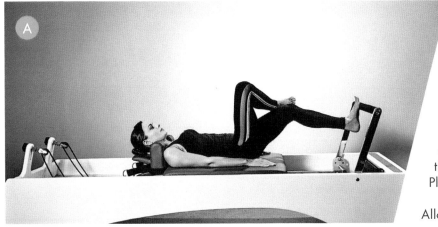

A & B. How to stretch

Press carriage away, bend knee and place ankle onto opposite thigh. Pelvis must remain neutral. Place hand under low back to assist.

Allow carriage to return to POT.

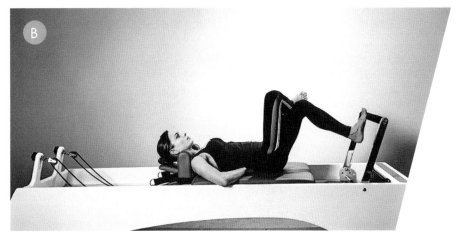

B. How to contract

Press ankle into thigh.

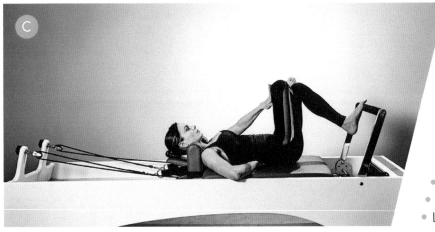

C. How to restretch

Allow carriage to move further toward foot bar.
Press knee of stretching leg away.

What to watch out for:

- Low back flattening.
- Bottom lifting/posterior pelvic rotation.
- Lateral pelvic rotation.

Seated External Hip Rotators

- **Standard:** Beginner/Intermediate/Advanced • **Spring Tension:** Heavy
- **Muscle Emphasis:** Gluteal group particularly deep hip rotators

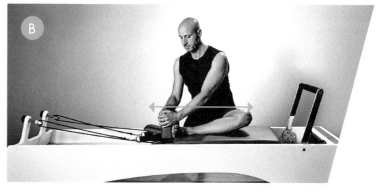

A & D. How to stretch

Sit and place leg across carriage with foot against opposite shoulder rest.
Stretch out rear leg.
Square hips to line of rear leg.
Level pelvis horizontally (for many this is a stretch in itself).

A. How to contract

Press ankle down into carriage.

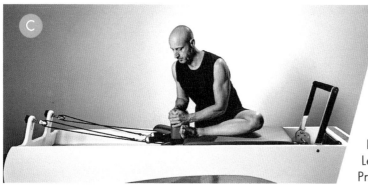

B & C. How to restretch

Lift chest and incline trunk forwards.
Lean breast bone/sternum toward foot.
Press rear leg away further to tilt pelvis anteriorly.

What to watch out for:

- Low back flattening.
- Spine bending/flexing.
- Hips not level horizontally.
- Hips not square.

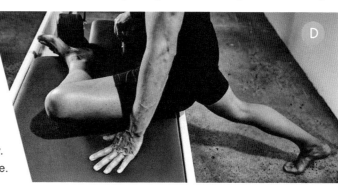

Seated Gluteals

- **Standard:** Beginner/Intermediate/Advanced • **Spring Tension:** Heavy
- **Muscle Emphasis:** Gluteal group particularly gluteus maximus

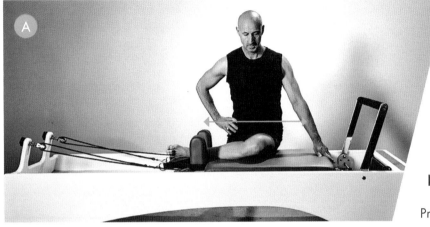

A & B. How to stretch

Place leg across carriage with foot on head rest.
Line up knee and navel.
Rotate/square hips to line of rear leg. Level pelvis horizontally. If position A is not much of a stretch, continue to position B.

B. How to contract

Press leg down into carriage.

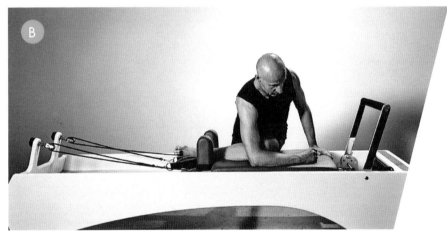

B. How to restretch

Incline trunk forwards.
Take armpit toward opposite knee.
Rotate pelvis/square hips to line of rear leg maximally.

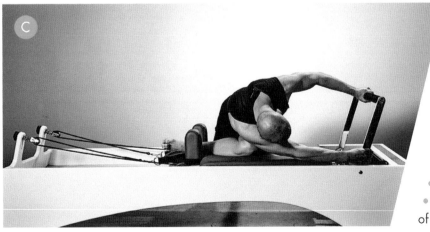

C. Advanced

Reach bottom arm to hold and pull on footbar.
Press top arm into sidebar.

What to watch out for:

- Hips not level horizontally.
- Hips not square.
- Rotation through thorax instead of pelvis.

The **maximus muscle** lies over the top of some of the medius muscle and obscures the six deep lateral rotators completely.

▼

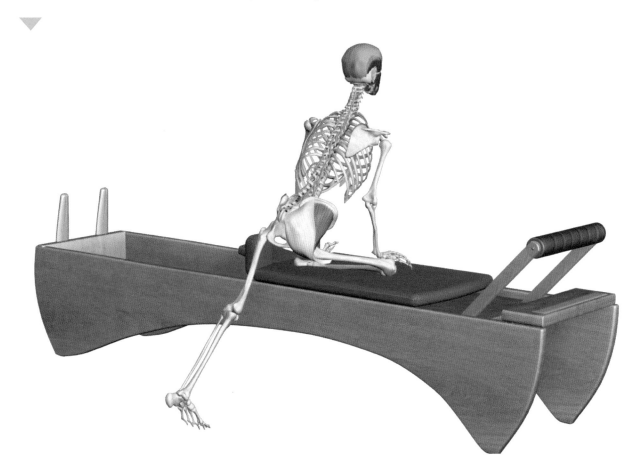

Note the deep muscles of the trunk, the multifidus, working to stabilise the relationship between spinal segments, or vertebrae.

The Pigeon Pose

- **Standard:** Advanced • **Spring Tension:** Medium
- **Muscle Emphasis:** Gluteal group particularly deep hip rotators

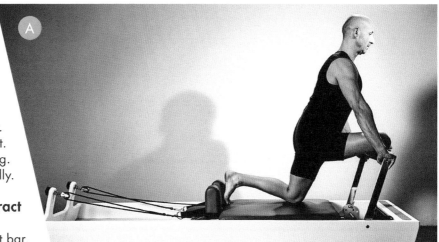

A & B. How to stretch

Place leg across foot bar.
Place rear foot against shoulder rest.
Square hips to line of rear leg.
Level pelvis horizontally.

How to contract

Press ankle down into foot bar.

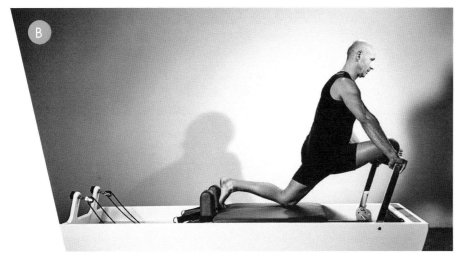

B. How to restretch

Lower hips below bar height.
Press rear leg away further.

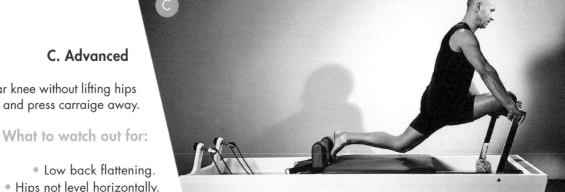

C. Advanced

Raise rear knee without lifting hips
and press carraige away.

What to watch out for:

- Low back flattening.
- Hips not level horizontally.
- Hips not square.

The gluteus medius, minimus, piriformis and obturator internus all insert onto the greater trochanter. When you flex and externally rotate the hip/femur and lean away from it, you will surely feel the stretch in all of them. ▶

Chapter Five

Adductors

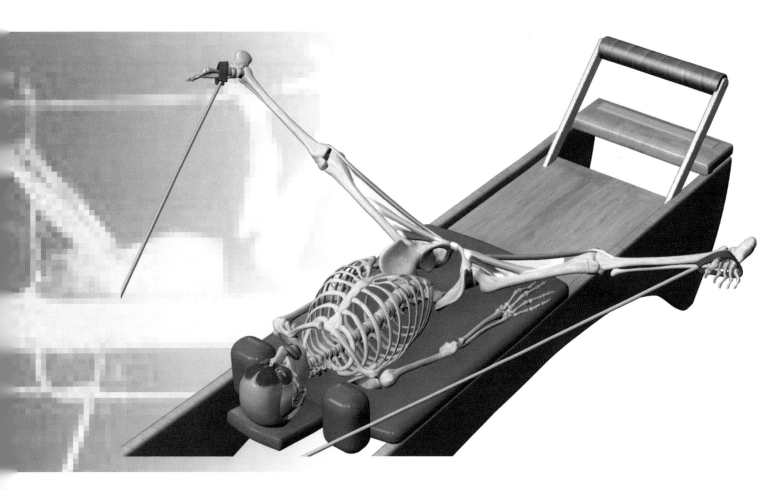

About the Adductors

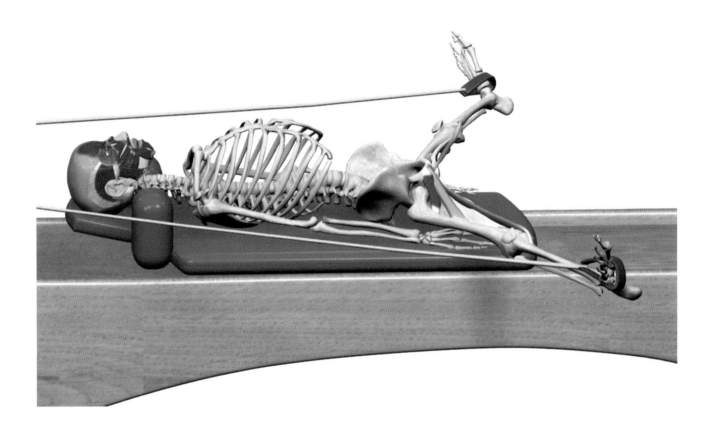

The line of force of the adductors approaches the hip from many different orientations. There are at least five primary adductors and three more "secondary adductors". "Secondary" muscles are those whose line of pull at various joint positions can assist in the primary action. This variation in orientation gives them a utilitarian function. At various hip joint angles they can extend the hip; at others they can assist in flexion.

It also means that to stretch all of them you need to explore various pelvic and femoral angles, so that all of their fibres are effectively stretched. You will notice that many of the stretches in this chapter have explorations and variations for this reason. Try them and, as always, work on the most difficult ones!

The Lying Splits

- **Standard:** Any • **Spring Tension:** Medium
- **Muscle Emphasis:** Entire adductor group and medial hamstrings

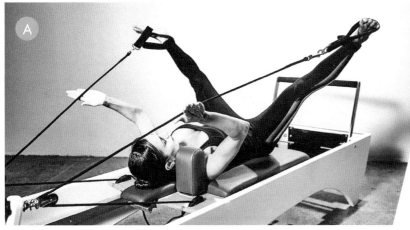

A. How to stretch

Take legs to 90 degrees from floor. Hold straps to enable legs to slowly come apart to POT.

Release straps from hands if comfortable (not shown).

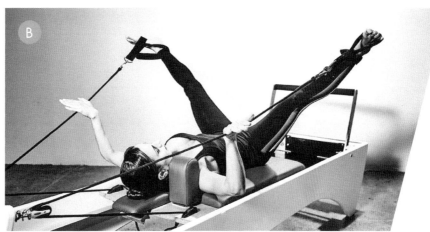

B. How to contract

Press legs back together and prevent any movement with hands.

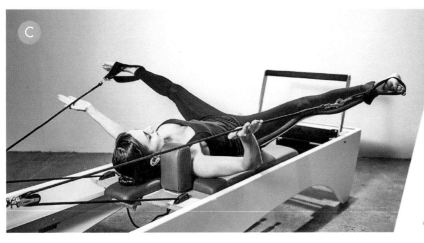

C. How to restretch

Allow legs to fall further apart. Use arms to press down onto straps for greater effect.

What to watch out for:

- Legs not at 90 degrees to begin.
- Not allowing legs to relax.
- Moving into stretch too quickly.

As the leg moves into more flexion (i.e. the feet moving toward the back end of the reformer), the posterior adductors like adductor magnus are stretched more strongly. Gracilis is the longest adductor, acting on both the knee and hip joints.

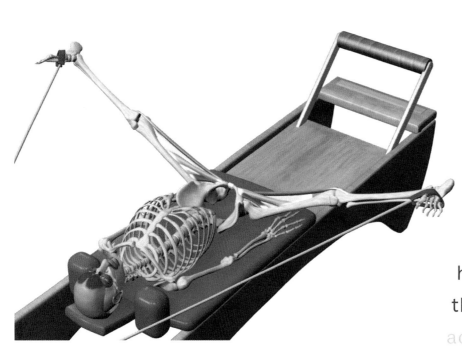

Topographically, the adductor muscles are organised into three layers. The most superficial layer can be seen here and includes the pectineus, adductor longus and gracilis.

Variations to Effect Different Adductors

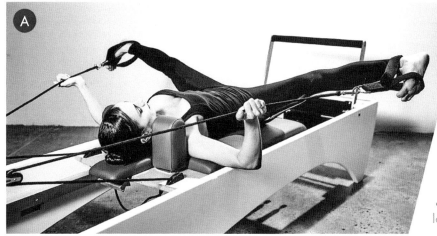

A. Externally rotate the legs for posterior adductors: adductor magnus.

B. Internally rotate legs for anterior adductors: pectineus and adductor longus.

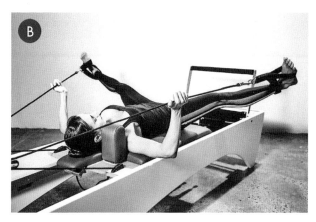

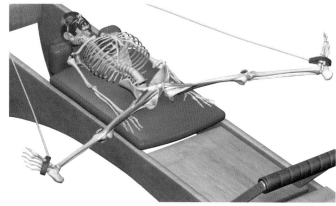

Variation Two

For muscle imbalances, bend one knee and allow the stretch to be felt mostly in the straight leg.

Straight leg can be taken into more or fewer degrees of hip flexion depending on sensations and requirements.

Greater hip flexion will translate to more effects on hamstrings and posterior adductors. See images above.

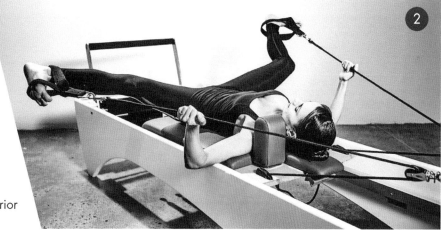

The Lying Splits From 45 Degrees

- Standard: Any • Spring Tension: Medium
- Muscle Emphasis: Anterior adductors and hip flexors

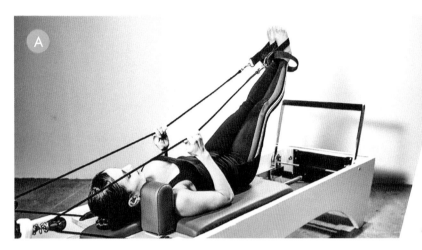

A & B. How to stretch

Take legs to 45 degrees from floor.
Hold straps to enable legs to slowly
come apart to POT.
Release straps from hands if
comfortable (not shown).

B. How to contract
*(Not shown. See
"Lying side slits from 90 degrees")*

Press legs back together. Press
legs up into hands (hip flexion not
shown).

B & C. How to restretch

Allow legs to fall further apart and
down toward floor. Use arms to press
down onto straps for greater effect.

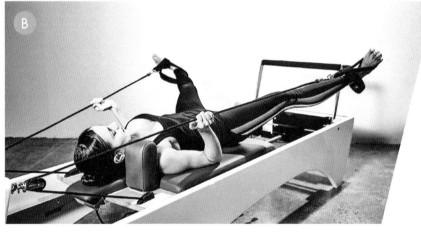

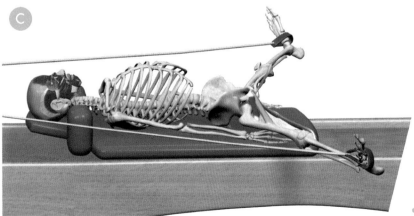

What to watch out for:

- Legs not at 45 degrees to begin.
- Allowing legs to creep up
  toward 90 degree of hip flexion.
- Not allowing legs to relax.
- Moving into stretch too quickly.

Try this!

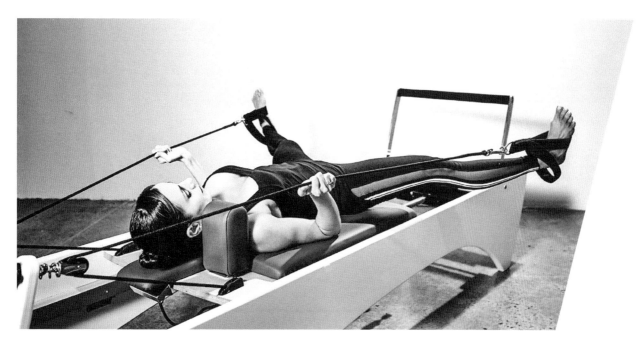

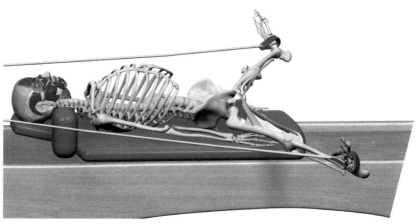

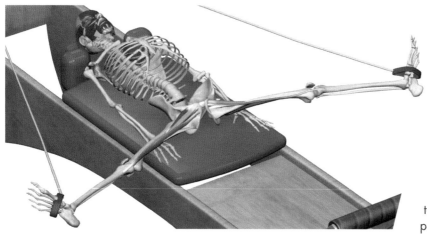

Internally rotate legs and lower feet toward floor for greater effect in pectineus and adductor longus.

The Standing Short Long

- **Standard:** Any • **Spring Tension:** Light
- **Muscle Emphasis:** Entire adductor group and hamstrings

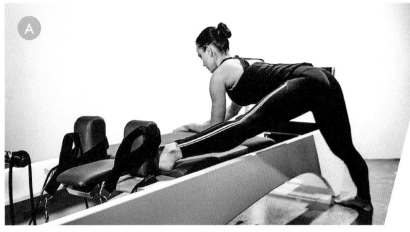

A & B. How to stretch

Press carriage away to POT in leg
on carriage (the stretching leg).
Then, slowly bend the knee
of the stance leg.
Support body weight with arms.

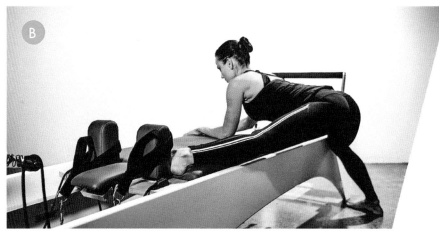

B. How to contract

Press foot on carriage
down into carriage.

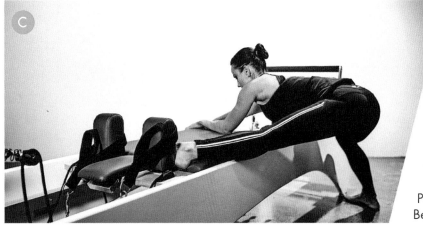

C. How to restretch

Press carriage away further.
Bend stance leg to lower hips.

Variations

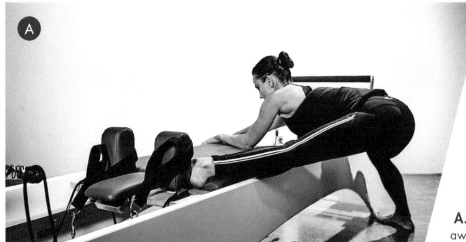

A. Lean bottom backwards away from carriage.

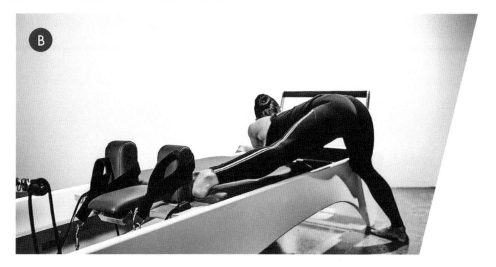

B. Turn chest right.

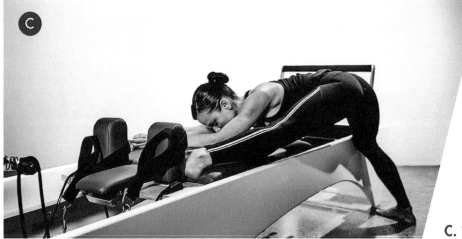

C. Turn chest left.

Hamstring Variation

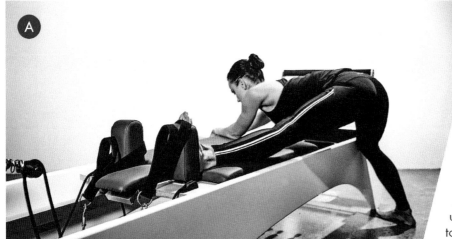

A. Turn leg and foot upwards (external rotation) to effect hamstrings.

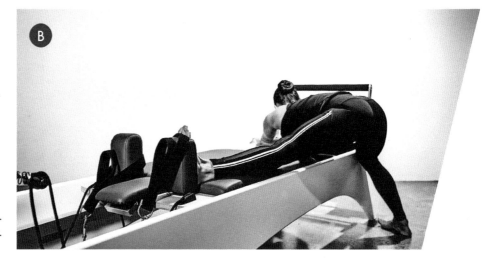

B. Lean bottom backwards. Turn chest right.

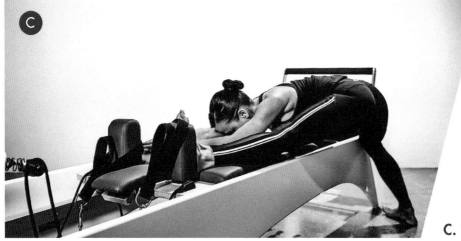

C. Turn chest left.

"Coming Home" Variation

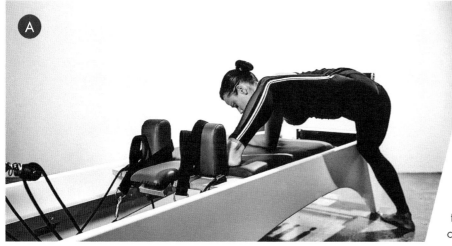

A. Return carriage by bending top knee. Place elbows onto carriage if possible.

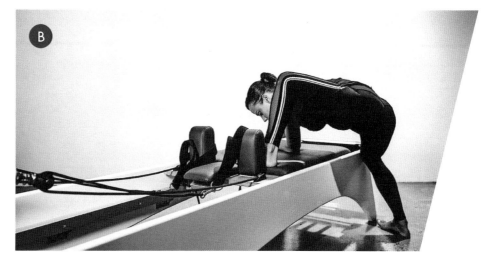

B. Lower chest inside thigh.

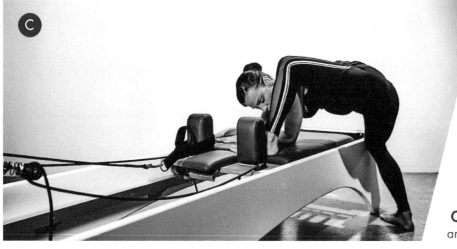

C. Lower chest and turn toward top foot.

The Squashed Frog

- Standard: Any • Spring Tension: Light
- Muscle Emphasis: Adductors

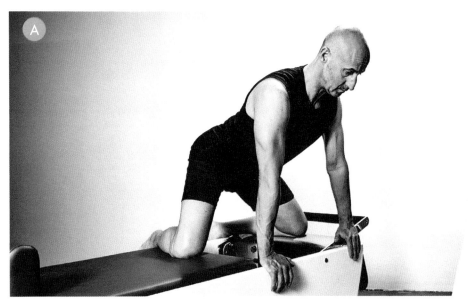

A. How to stretch

Kneel on reformer, hips in line with knees. Take carriage (abduct legs) away to POT.
You can arms and legs to move carriage.

A. How to contract: Press legs back together.

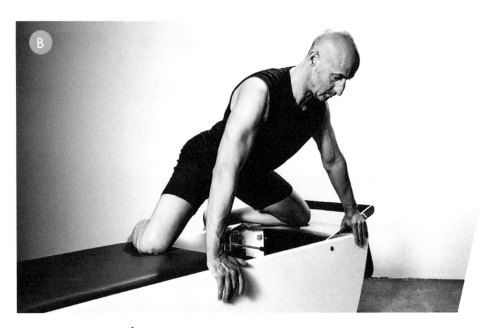

B. How to restretch
Allow knees/legs to slide further apart and lower hips.
Use arms to assist with holding carriage and supporting body weight.

Variations

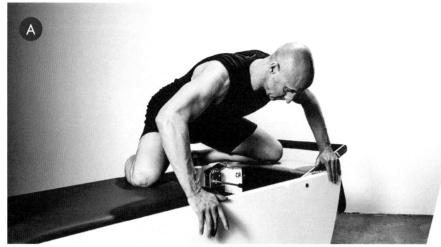

A. Lean hips backward and forward.

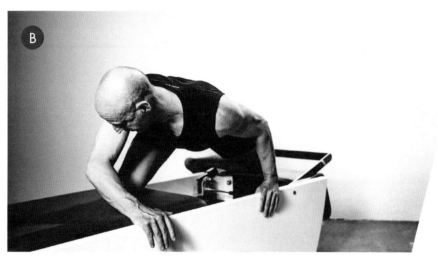

B. Twist right and hold.

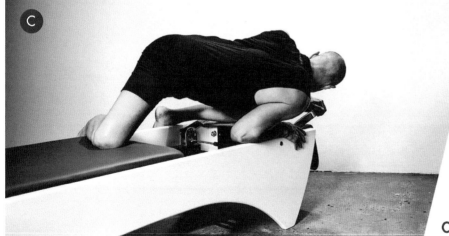

C. Twist left and hold.

Chapter Six

The Spine

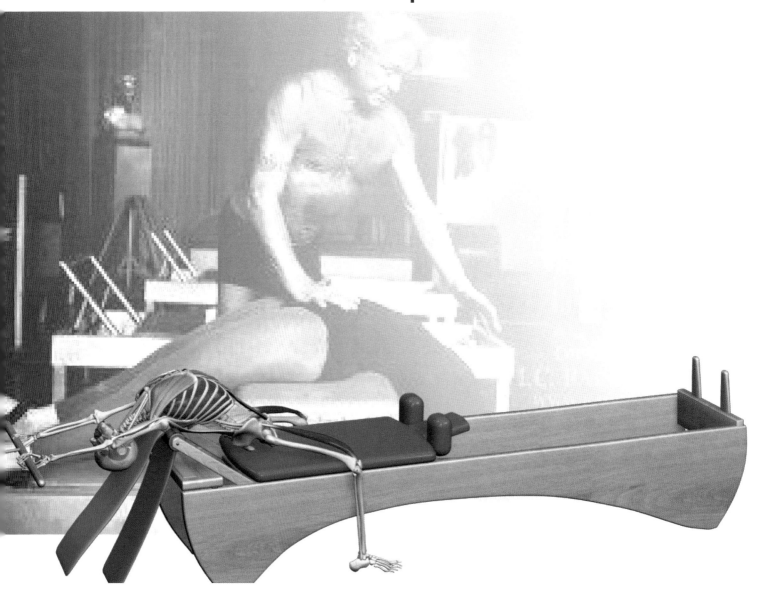

About this Chapter

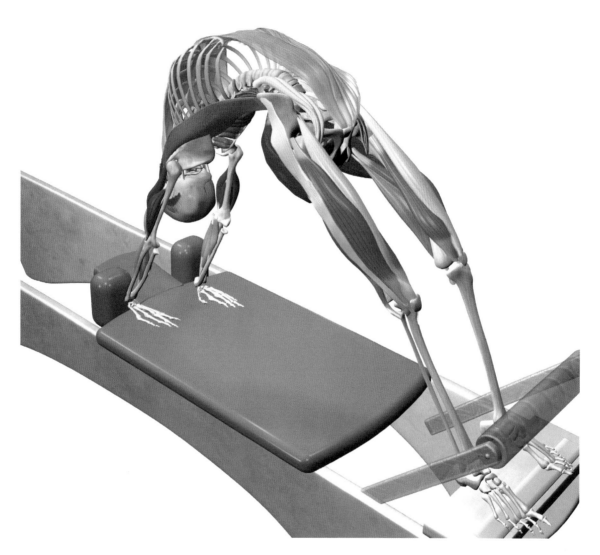

This chapter is divided into the movements of the spine. There is flexion or forward bending – and its opposite, extension or backbending – rotation or twisting, and lateral flexion or side bending. These and their combinations are the essential movements of daily living, and must be maintained for a healthy spine.

Within each section there are beginners to advanced stretches. Ensure that, in your practice, you include at least one stretch from each section.

Flexion

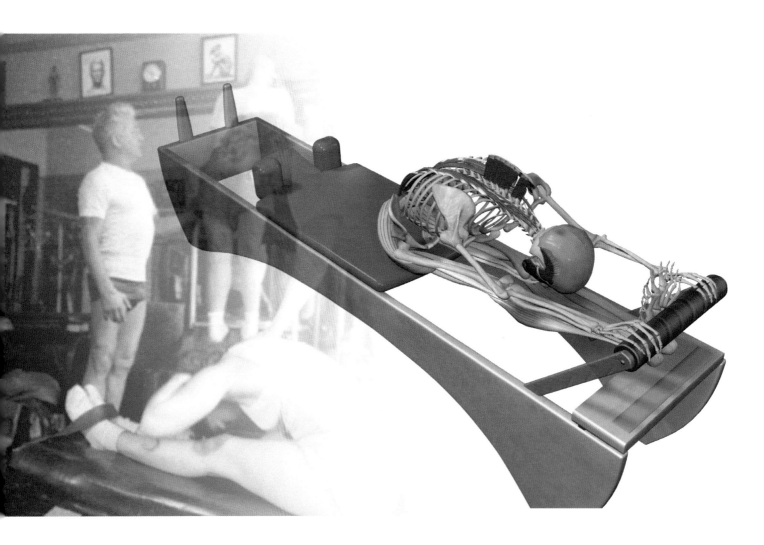

Flexion/the Reverse Curl

- **Standard:** Any • **Spring Tension:** Medium
- **Muscle Emphasis:** All spinal extensors from superficial to deep. levator scapula, upper trapezius, rhomboids, splenius

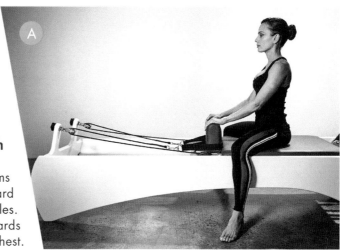

A & B. How to stretch

Sit with hands on shoulder rests, arms slightly bent. Slump or roll pelvis backward (posterior tilt). Tighten abdominal muscles. Press arms away and upwards into shoulder rests. Take chin toward chest.

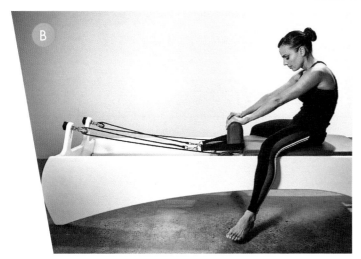

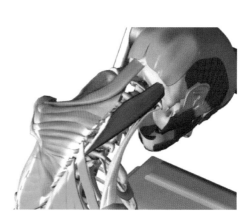

C. Variations

Tilt (laterally flex) and rotate head to both shoulders (levator scapula, upper trapezius).

What to watch out for:

- Not enough pelvic tilt.
- Not pressing arms upward.
- Not tilting head laterally.

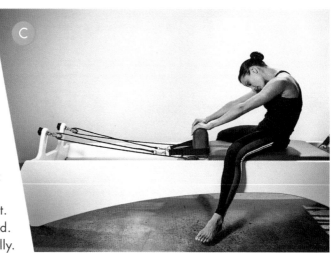

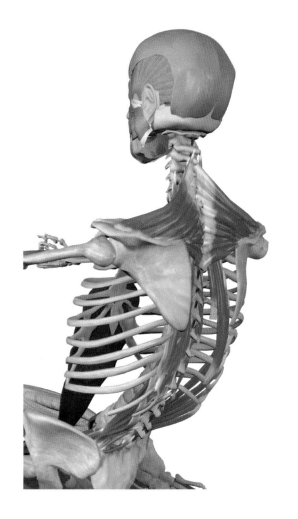

Erector spinae and mid trapezius will stretch as the trunk flexes and the shoulder blades move apart, known as "protraction".

Contract abdominals To deepen the flexion of the trunk and increase the posterior pelvic tilt. The psoas minor may also assist with this action.

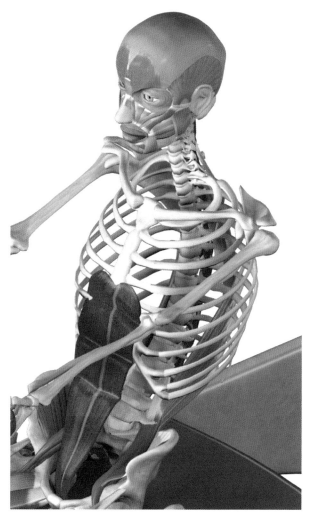

The Posterior Stretch

- **Standard:** Beginner • **Spring Tension:** Light - Medium
- **Muscle Emphasis:** All spinal extensors from superficial to deep, hamstrings, calves, adductor magnus, gluteus maximus, latissimus dorsi

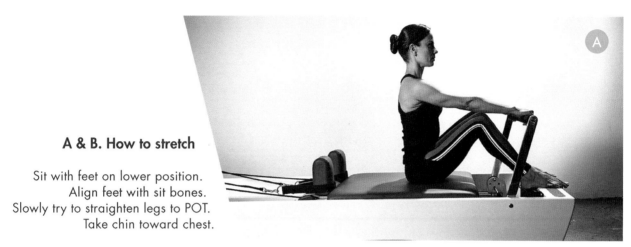

A & B. How to stretch

Sit with feet on lower position.
Align feet with sit bones.
Slowly try to straighten legs to POT.
Take chin toward chest.

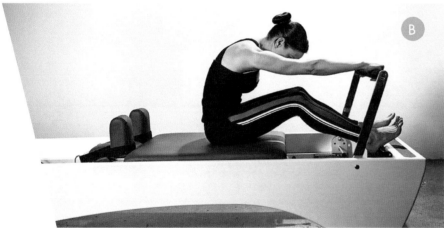

B. How to contract

Press feet down into reformer.

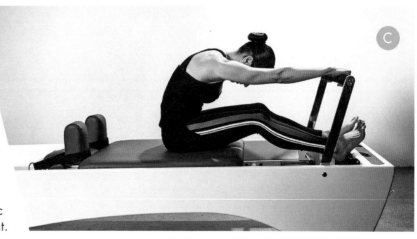

C. How to restretch

Straighten legs further.

What to watch out for:

- Moving carriage out too fast.
- Not taking chin to chest.
- Too much flexion in thoracic spine and legs still bent.

The Posterior Stretch 2.0

- **Standard:** Beginner • **Spring Tension:** Light - Medium
- **Muscle Emphasis:** All spinal extensors from superficial to deep, hamstrings, calves, adductor magnus, gluteus maximus, latissimus dorsi

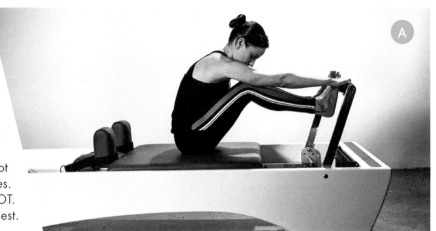

A & B. How to stretch

Sit with hands and balls of feet on foot bar. Align feet with sit bones. Slowly try to straighten legs to POT. Take chin toward chest.

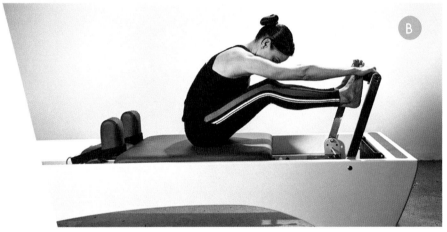

B. How to contract

Press feet down into foot bar. Try to lift chest to straighten spine.

C. How to restretch

Straighten legs fully if possible.

What to watch out for:

- Moving carriage out too fast.
  - Not taking chin to chest.
  - Too much flexion in thorax and legs still bent.

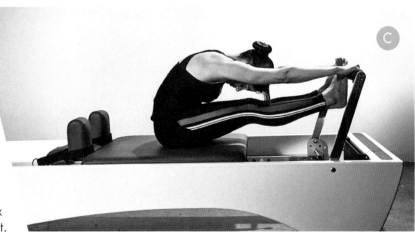

As you straighten your legs, the entire chain of muscles on the posterior surface of your body will stretch.

The calf group, the hamstrings and the entire erector spinae group will stretch. Because of the fascial interconnectedness of these groups, tension in one area can be transmitted to another region.

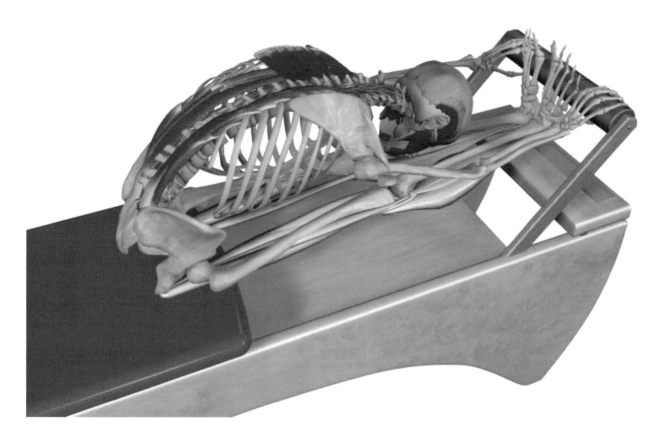

Note for teachers: Common postural compensation patterns associated with tightness in this posterior chain include ankle dorsiflexion restriction, knee hyperextension, hamstring shortness, sacral nutation, upper cervical hyperextension and rotation of the occiput.

The latissimus dorsi, a large and important muscle on the back and arms, will often be stretched here too.

In conjunction with the transverses abdominus, the latissimus can be used to safeguard your spine if you feel it is vulnerable during this stretch.

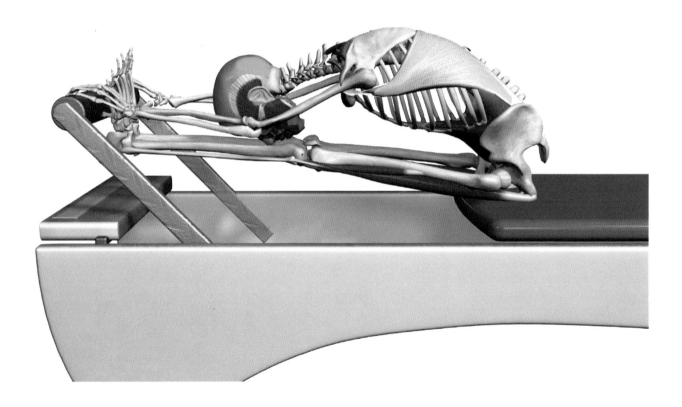

Please take our "Safeguarding the Spine" online workshop for tips and cues on integrating a greater strength element into this stretch.

 "Safeguarding the Spine" Workshop at www.innovationsinpilates.com

Because a portion of the large and powerful gluteus maximus attach onto the leg bone or femur, they will be stretched in this position also.

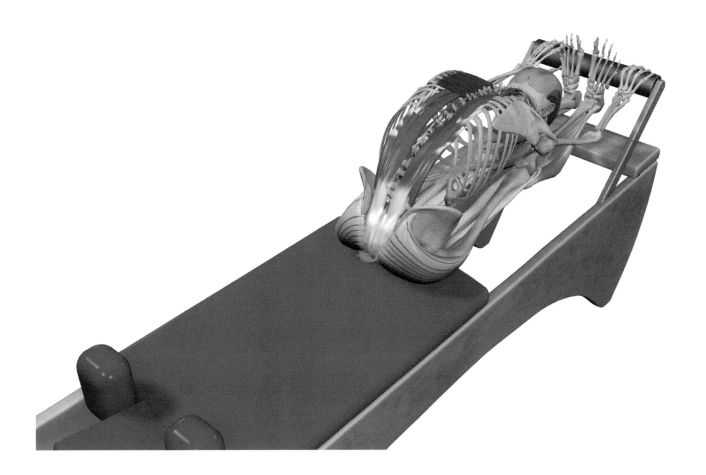

If you are tight, and your shoulder blades rotate upwardly, your rhomboids will also feel a degree of stretch.

The Posterior Stretch 3.0

- **Standard:** Advanced ● **Spring Tension:** Light - Medium
- **Muscle Emphasis:** All spinal extensors from superficial to deep, hamstrings, calves, adductor magnus, gluteus maximus, latissimus dorsi

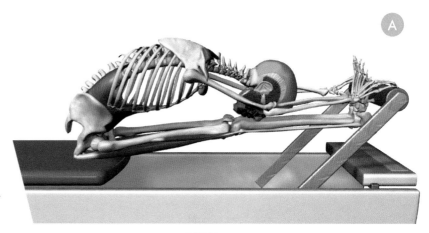

A. How to stretch

Slowly straighten legs to POT.
Take chin toward chest.

A. How to contract
Press feet down into foot bar.

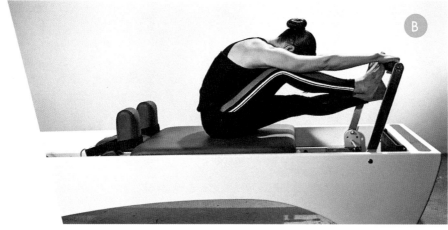

B & C. How to restretch

Lower one heel and bend other leg or lower both heels.

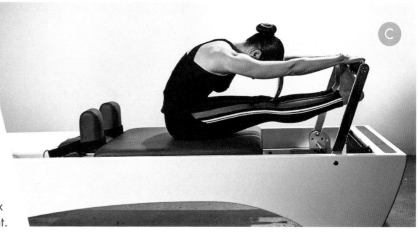

What to watch out for:

- Moving carriage out too fast.
  - Not taking chin to chest.
  - Too much flexion in thorax and legs still bent.

The Posterior Stretch 4.0

- **Standard:** Advanced • **Spring Tension:** Light - Medium
- **Muscle Emphasis:** Hamstrings, calves, adductor magnus, gluteus maximus

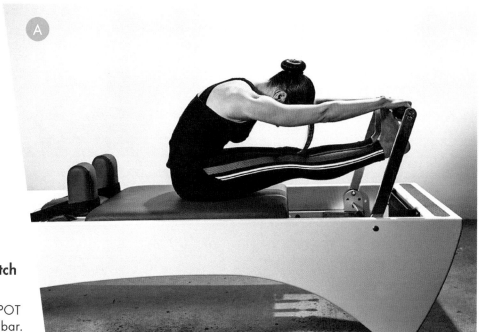

A. How to stretch

Slowly straighten legs to POT and lower heels under bar.

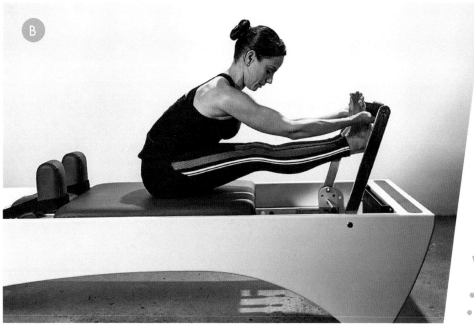

B. How to contract

Press feet down into foot bar. Try to lift chest to straighten spine.

B. How to restretch
Lower both heels further.
Arch spine backwards (extension).
Pull chest toward legs – see underhanded bar grip.

What to watch out for:

- Moving carriage out too fast.
- Allowing spine to flex/bend.

The Pull Push

- Standard: Any • Spring Tension: No Springs
- Muscle Emphasis: All spinal extensors, rhomboids, middle & upper trapezius, levato scapular

A. How to stretch

Sit on oblique angle to foot bar. Roll pelvis backward/ posteriorly strongly to ensure carriage does not move by sending pubic bone toward foot bar. Place hands on bar as pictured. Pull lightly with arm on sidebar. Push strongly with arm into foot bar. Take chin toward chest. Lean whole body backwards strongly.

A. How to contract

Pull on sidebar with arm trying to retract scapula.

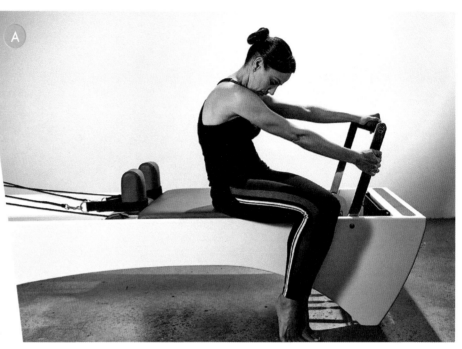

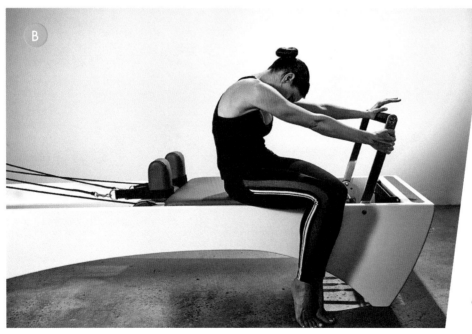

B. How to restretch
Lean back further.
Tighten abdominal muscles.
Tilt ear toward top (left in photo) arm.

What to watch out for:

- Carriage moving out.
- Not taking chin to chest.
- Not leaning backwards.
- Not thrusting pelvis toward footbar.

The middle and upper trapezius muscles will stretch, along with the rhomboids; mostly on the side with the arm on the side bar. Be sure to swap and do both sides.

As you take your chin toward your chest, your levator scapula and splenius capitis muscles will also be stretched.

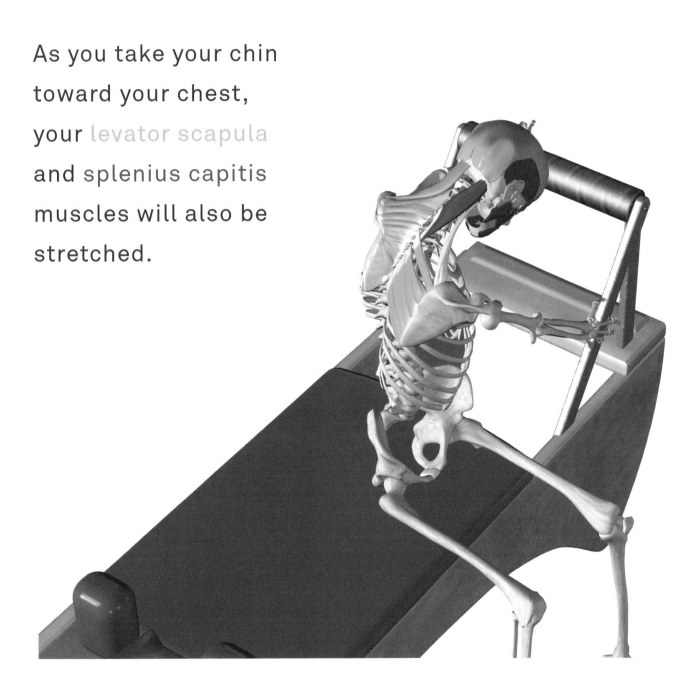

The Dangler

- **Standard:** Any • **Spring Tension:** Heavy
- **Muscle Emphasis:** Entire posterior spinal muscles, posterior disks, posterior portion of internal obliques, transversus abdominus, quadratus lumborum

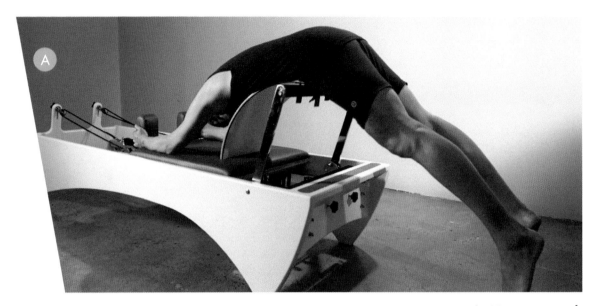

A. How to stretch
Clasp carriage and then shoulder rests as pictured. Allow legs to hang or dangle. Hold for 90 seconds.

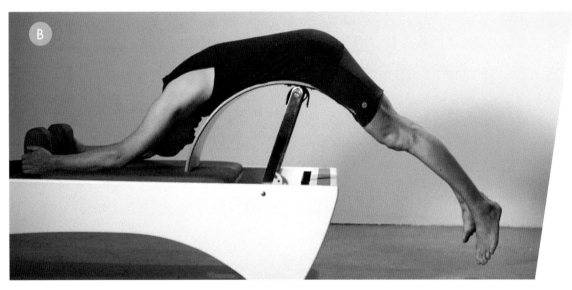

How to breathe
Take deep abdominal breaths to expand abdominal region.

What to watch out for:
- Lifting head or feet, which engages spinal muscles.
- Shallow breathing.
- Coming out of the stretch too quickly.

Rotation

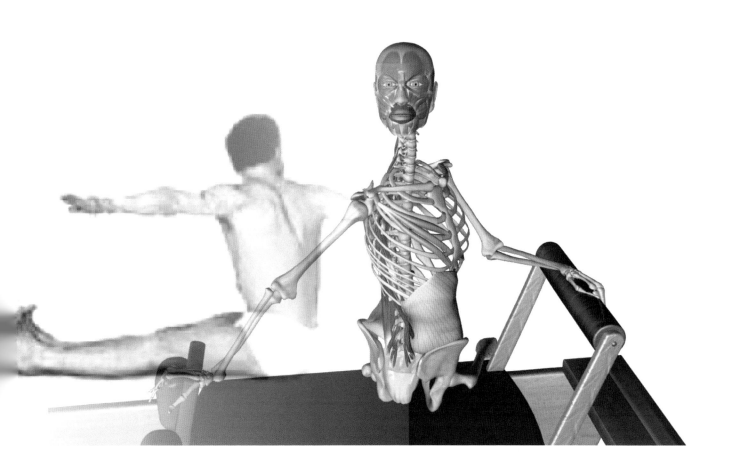

Reaching Under the Table

- **Standard:** Intermediate/Advanced • **Spring Tension:** Heavy
- **Muscle Emphasis:** Rhomboids, middle trapezius, oblique abdominals, posterior deltoids

A & B. How to stretch

Kneel on carriage parallel to foot bar just over arms-length away. Ensure hips are above knees. Ensure carriage does not move. Reach under with outside arm to clasp low bar. Lower chest and shoulder. Reach with other arm/top arm to clasp footbar. Push strongly with top arm into foot bar. Lean whole body backwards strongly.

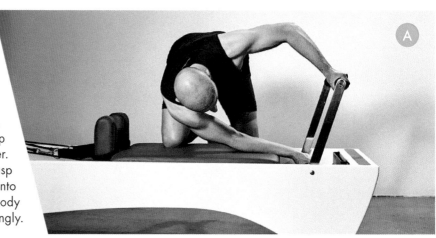

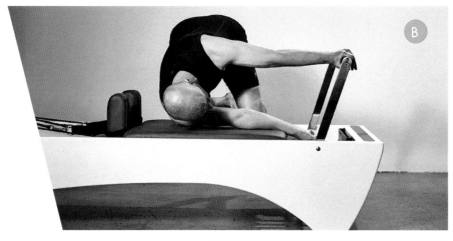

B. How to contract

Pull with lower hand and shoulder on lower bar, trying to retract scapula.

C. How to restretch

Lean back further. Straighten top arm if possible. Shift bar to vertical position if possible.

What to watch out for:

- Carriage moving out.
- Not leaning backwards.
- Not lowering chest &and shoulder to carriage.

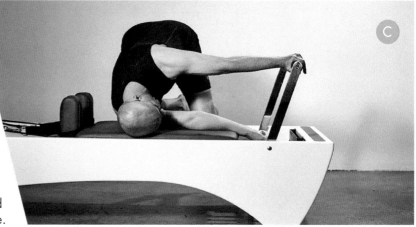

The Seated Rotation

- **Standard**: Any • **Spring Tension**: Heavy
- **Muscle Emphasis**: Oblique abdominals, intercostals, deep spinal rotators, spinal joints and disks

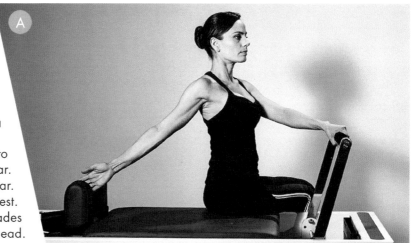

A & B. How to stretch

Sit on carriage on oblique angle to foot bar. Leg against foot bar. Pull with arm on foot bar. Push with arm on shoulder rest. Lift chest and draw shoulder blades together. Rotate head.

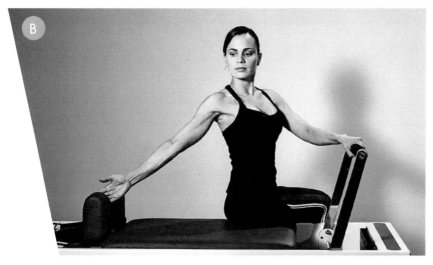

B. How to contract

Try to twist back toward start position using abdominal muscles.

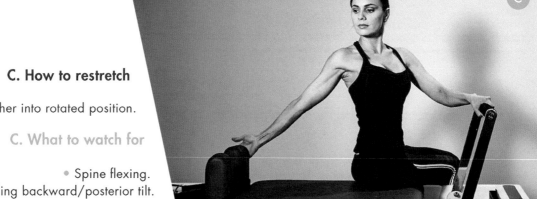

C. How to restretch

Twist further into rotated position.

C. What to watch for

- Spine flexing.
- Pelvis rolling backward/posterior tilt.
- Shallow breathing.

The external oblique will stretch, in particular if you exaggerate your breathing to expand the abdominal cavity.

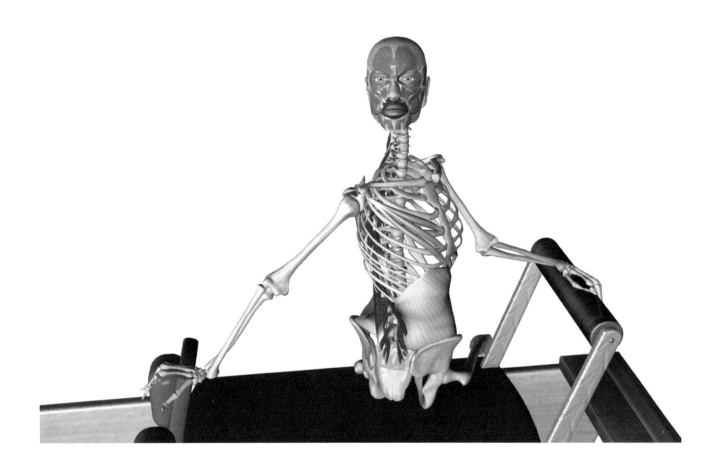

The spinal extensors will work strongly to keep you sitting up straight.

The pectoralis minor will assist in breathing by lifting the rib cage.

The middle and lower trapezius muscles work strongly to retract (draw together) and depress the scapula. This opens the chest, and enables pectoralis minor to lift the anterior chest wall.

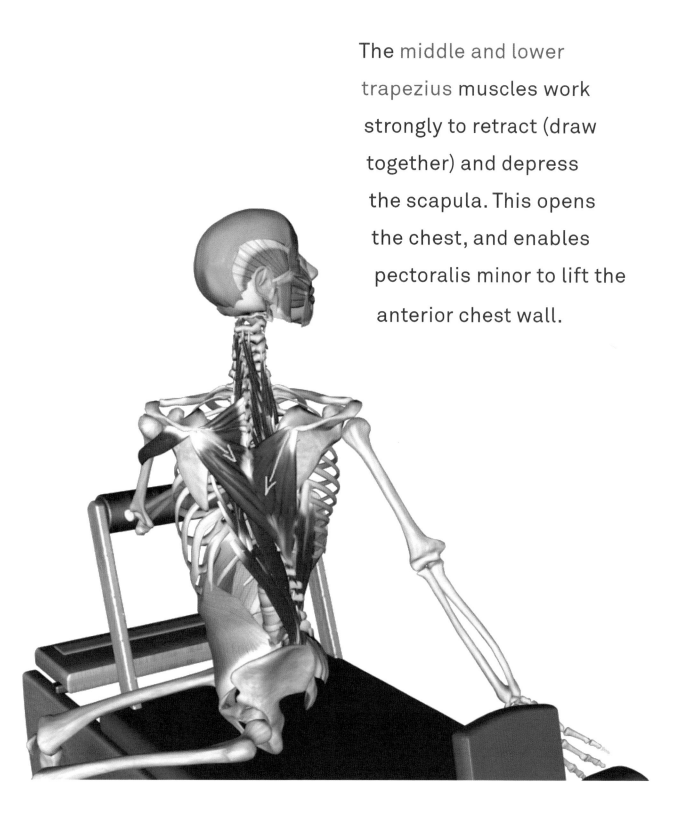

Lying Rotation

- **Standard:** Any • **Spring Tension:** Heavy
- **Muscle Emphasis:** Pectorals, anterior deltoid, serratus anterior, spinal extensors, oblique abdominals, gluteal group, abductors

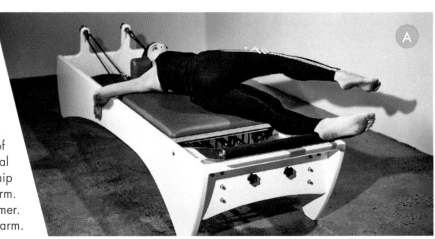

A. How to stretch

Hook hand under or onto side of reformer and lower the elbow. Move opposite hip bone to centre of carriage to maintain spinal alignment/elongation. Rotate hip and leg away from top arm. Drape leg over side of reformer. Press down on leg with free arm.

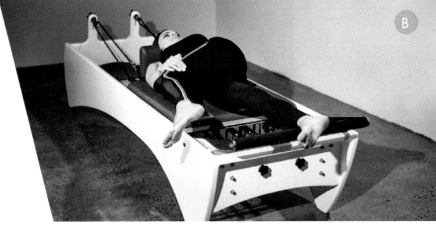

B. How to contract

Press arm up into reformer. Press top leg back into free arm.

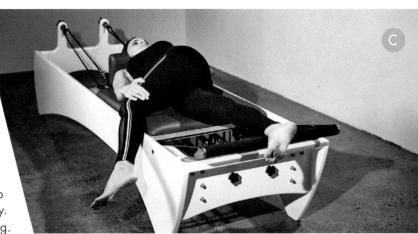

C. How to restretch

Twist further into rotated position. Press bent knee down.

What to watch out for:

- Not shifting hip to center of carriage initially.
- Shallow breathing.

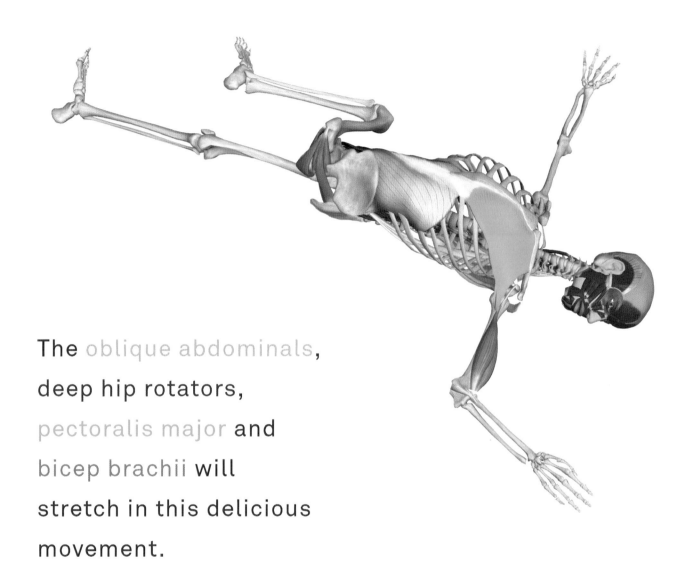

The oblique abdominals, deep hip rotators, pectoralis major and bicep brachii will stretch in this delicious movement.

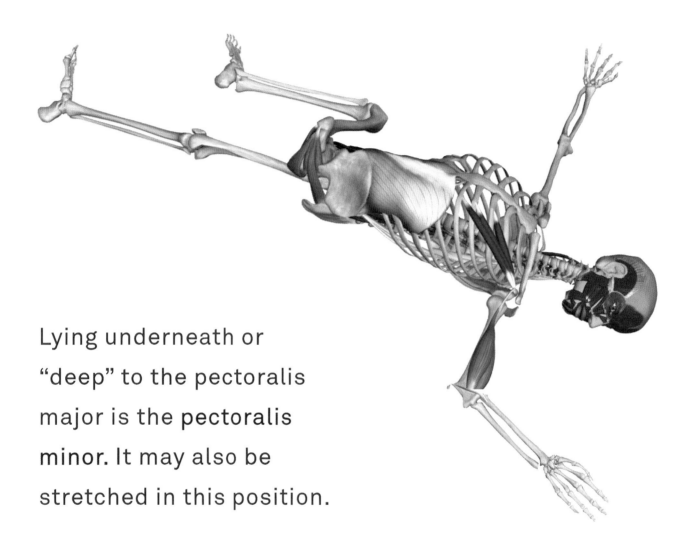

Lying underneath or
"deep" to the pectoralis
major is the pectoralis
minor. It may also be
stretched in this position.

"We live in a kyphotic age"
Lolita San Miguel, 2015

Extension

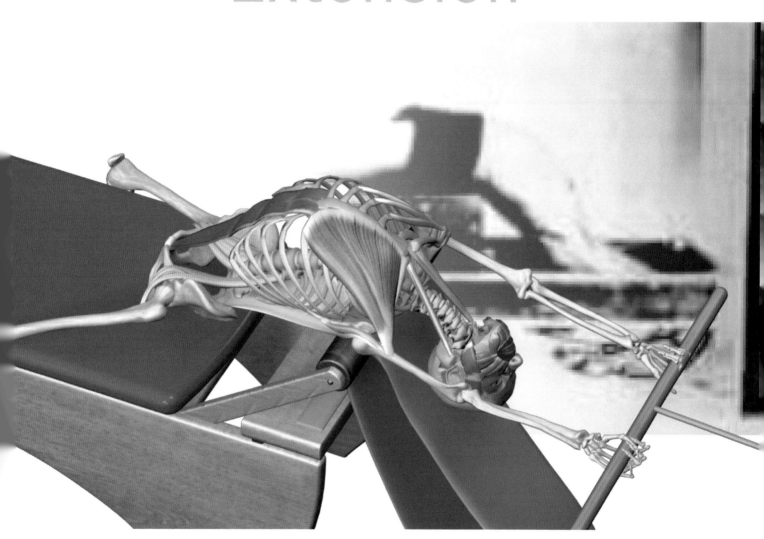

Chest Press

- **Standard:** Any • **Spring Tension:** Heavy
- **Muscle Emphasis:** Pectorals, latissimus dorsi, triceps-long head, thoracic joints, rectus abdominus

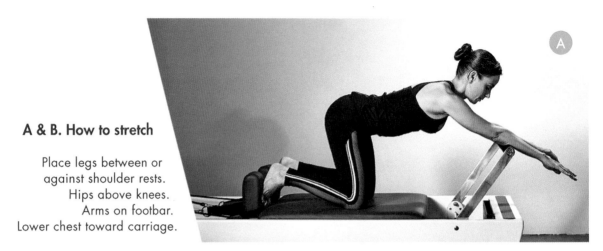

A & B. How to stretch

Place legs between or
against shoulder rests.
Hips above knees.
Arms on footbar.
Lower chest toward carriage.

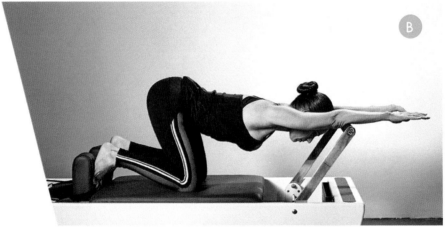

B. How to contract

Press arms down into footbar.

C. How to restretch

Lower chest further
toward carriage.

What to watch out for:

- Hips not above knees.
- Shoulder pain/impingement.
  (If shoulder pain occurs,
  see alternate arm position.)

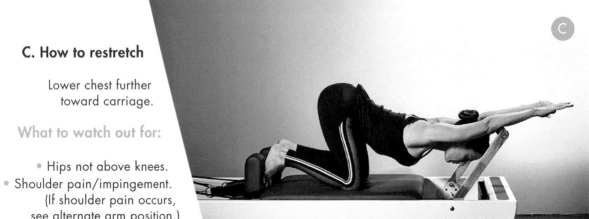

Variation One

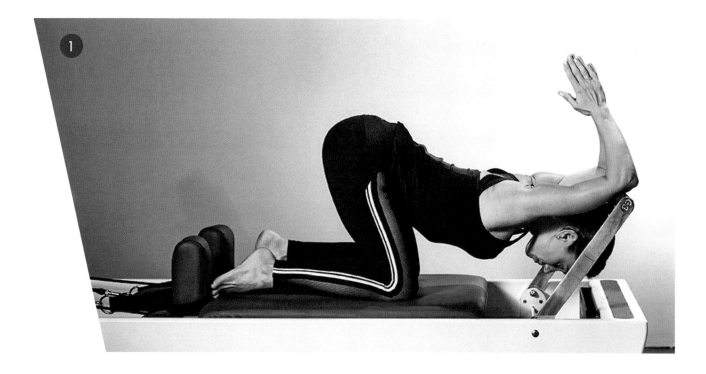

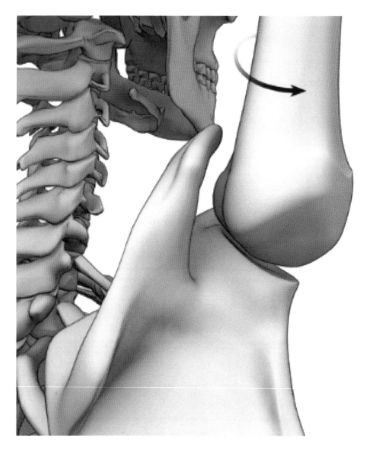

External rotation will create space under the shoulder bone/acromiom to alleviate painful joint impingement.

Variation Two

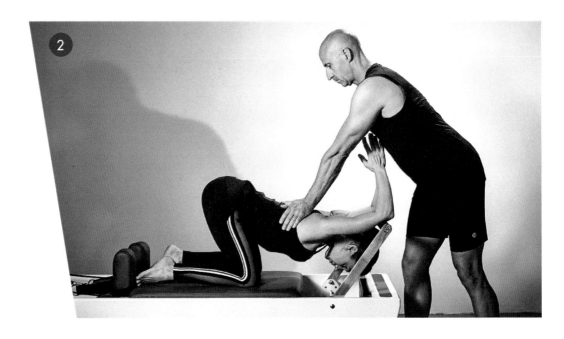

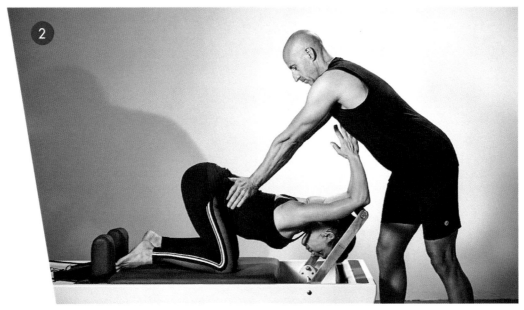

Partner can press on spine, starting between shoulder blades and working toward low back.

The Cobra

- **Standard:** Any • **Spring Tension:** Light - Medium
- **Muscle Emphasis:** Abdominals, anterior surface of disks, hip flexors

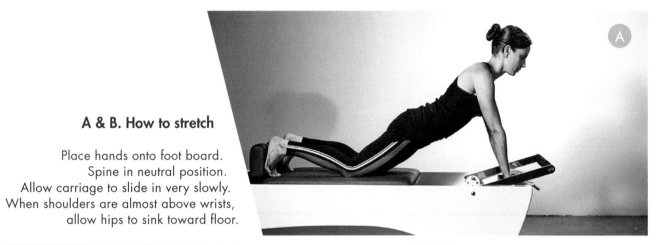

A & B. How to stretch

Place hands onto foot board.
Spine in neutral position.
Allow carriage to slide in very slowly.
When shoulders are almost above wrists,
allow hips to sink toward floor.

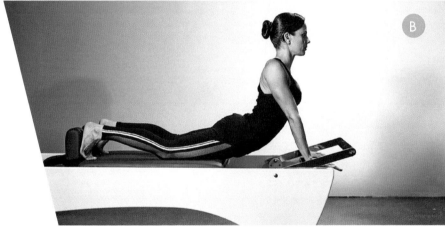

B. How to contract

Press hands and feet
downwards.

C. How to restretch

Lower hips further toward carriage/
floor. Relax all muscles including
shoulders and lats.Explore gently
rotating to both sides.

How to breathe
Deeply, filling entire abdominal region.

What to watch out for:
- Failure to allow low back
and gluteal muscles to relax.

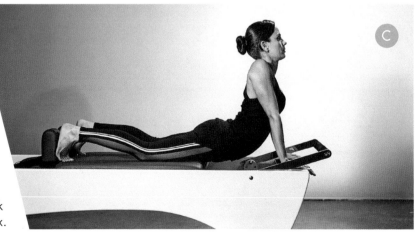

The Cobra 2.0

- **Standard:** Intermediate/Advanced • **Spring Tension:** Light - Medium
- **Muscle Emphasis:** Abdominals, anterior surface of disks, neck flexors, intrinsic foot muscles, hip flexors

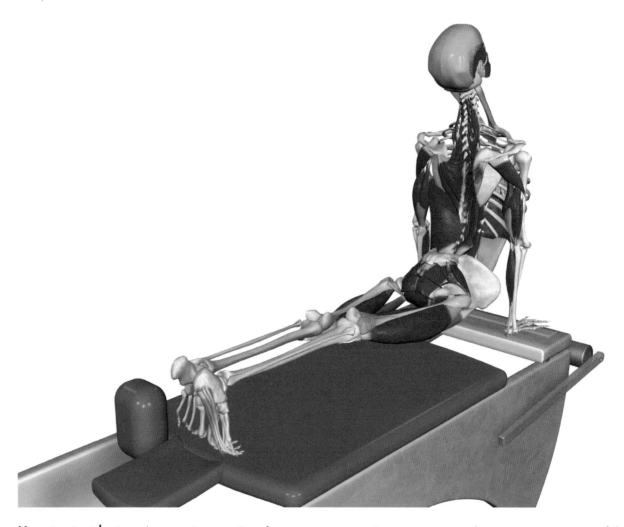

How to stretch: See photos in Version One for set-up position. Once in position, this version uses some of the posterior extensor muscles to deepen the anterior stretch. Contract the erector spinae, **mid and** lower trapezius muscles to arch the spine backwards. Try to keep the gluteal muscles relaxed to maximise the lumbar extension. Take your head back if comfortable also. Explore moving the carriage in or out a fraction.

How to breath

Deeply, filling entire abdominal region.
Hold for 30 to 60 seconds.

What to watch out for:
- Failure to allow gluteal muscles to relax.

The Cobra 3.0

- **Standard:** Intermediate/Advanced • **Spring Tension:** Medium
- **Muscle Emphasis:** Abdominals, anterior surface of disks, hip flexors

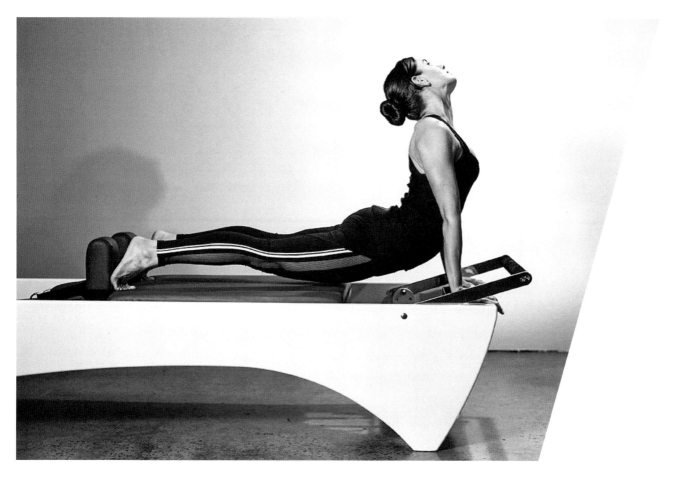

How to Stretch: Follow the set-up instructions for V1 and V2. Once in position, contract the quadriceps muscles to lift the knees. This will deepen the stretch and add a further strength dimension. Tilt head back and to the side slowly.

Major differences

Tilt head laterally to both sides.
Lift knees to straighten legs.

How to breath

Deeply, filling entire abdominal region.
Hold for 30 to 60 seconds.

The quadriceps will contract to straighten the legs. As a result, the rectus femoris will pull the pelvis forward/anteriorly, deepening the stretch.

The illiopsoas may stretch. The diaphragm can be strengthened by deep inhalations. As it descends, it will encounter some resistance from the abdominal content. Maximising the inhalations will strengthen it against this resistance.

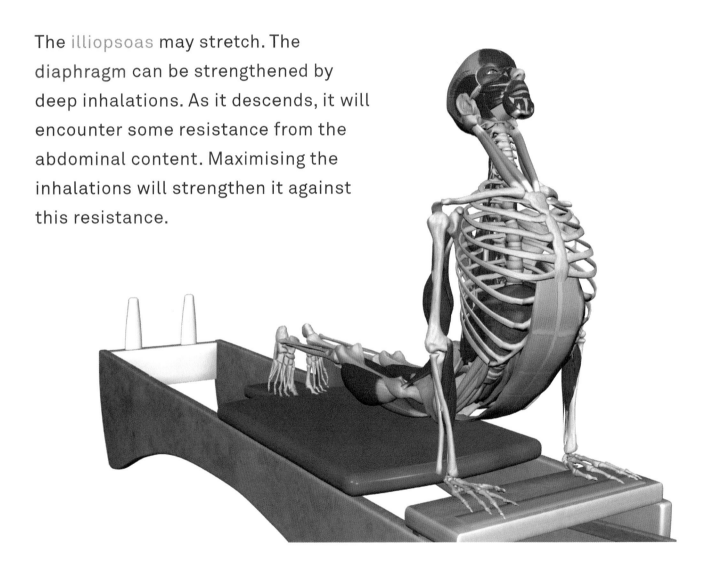

The abdominals will stretch as the diaphragm descends and distends the belly.

The sternocleidomastoid will stretch by taking the head backwards.

The High Bridge: Elevated Feet

- **Standard:** Advanced • **Spring Tension:** Medium to Heavy
- **Muscle Emphasis:** Hip Flexors, abdominals, pectorals, lats, anterior neck.
  NB. Elevated feet requires less bend in lumbar spine.

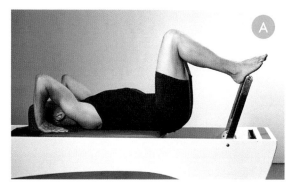

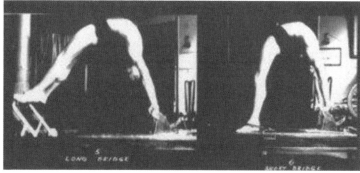

A, B & C. How to stretch

Lie on carriage, slide away a little from shoulder rests. Lift onto top of head. Lift/press up into full bridge.

C. How to contract

Press hands and feet away from each other.

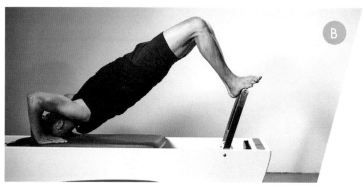

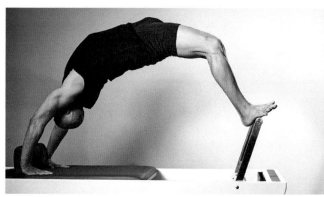

D. How to restretch

Allow carriage to move further toward footbar. Press away with legs a little to increase thoracic bend and shift shoulders over hands.

What to watch out for:

- Arms bending.
- Hips dropping.
- Legs/feet not staying parallel.

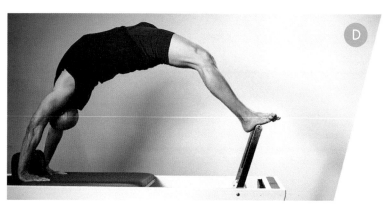

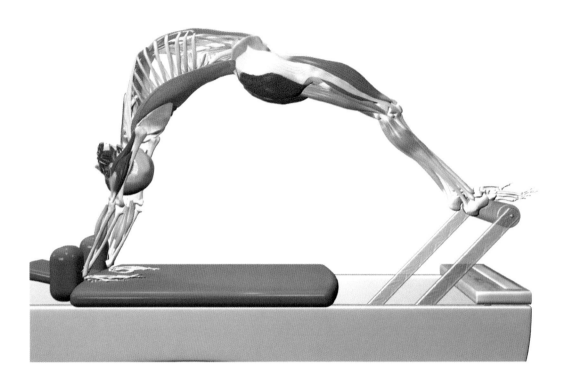

This is an intense stretch and strength exercise. The muscles on the inside of the curve work hard to lift and then maintain the position. You can see the hamstrings, gluteus maximus, and triceps contracting. On the outside of the curve, on the front of the body, the _____, rectus femoris, rectus abdominus and pectoralis major are stretched.

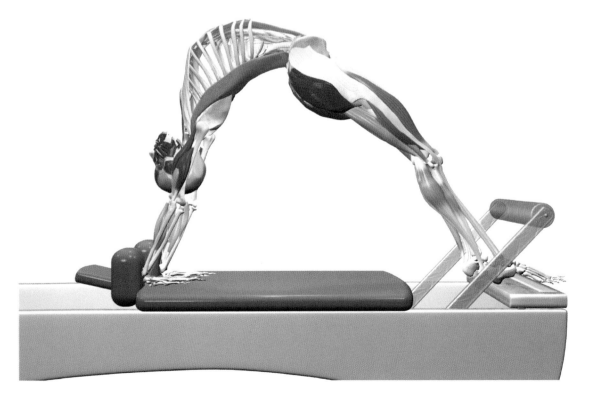

The High Bridge 2.0

- **Standard:** Advanced • **Spring Tension:** Medium to Heavy
- **Muscle Emphasis:** Hip flexors, abdominals, pectorals, lats, anterior neck
  NB. Lowering feet results in more bend in lumbar spine.

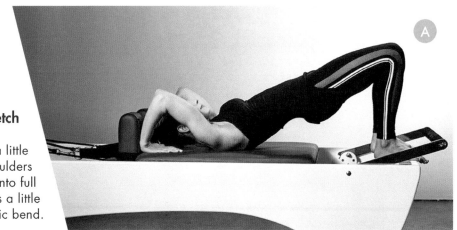

A & B. How to stretch

Lie on carriage, slide away a little from shoulder rests. Lift onto shoulders or top of head. Lift/press up into full bridge. Straighten legs a little to increase thoracic bend.

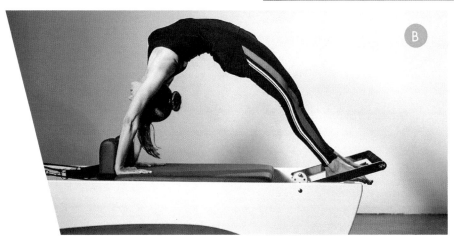

B. How to contract

Press hands and feet away from each other.

How to restretch

Allow carriage to move further toward footbar.

What to watch out for:

- Arms bending.
- Hips dropping.

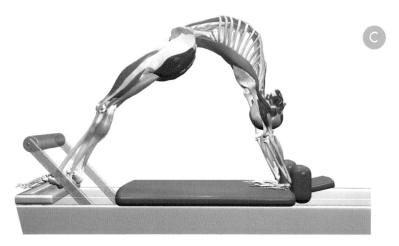

Seated Backbend

- **Standard:** Beginner/Intermediate • **Spring Tension:** Heavy
- **Muscle Emphasis:** Psoas, rectus femoris, abdominals, pectorals, lats, anterior neck, triceps long head, rotator cuff

How to stretch

Place secure box close to foot bar to support head.
Sit on carriage close to footbar.
Sit back so that bar is just below scapula/shoulder blades.
Take hands and head back slowly.

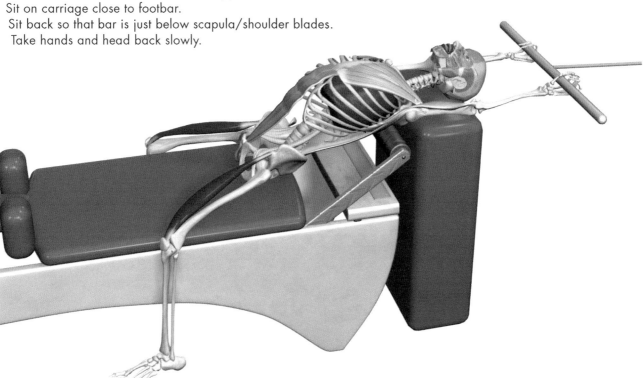

How to contract

Press hands and thighs up toward ceiling.

How to restretch

Allow pelvis, legs and arms to drop/flop.
Partner can pull arms downward and alternately pull one side more.

What to watch out for:

- Unnecessary tension in arms, neck, stomach.
- Dizziness is a strong sign to stop immediately.

Seated Backbend 2.0

- **Standard:** Intermediate/Advanced • **Spring Tension:** Heavy
- **Muscle Emphasis:** Psoas, abdominals, pectoralis major, pectoralis minor, lats, triceps long head, rotator cuff

How to stretch

Sit on carriage close to footbar.
Sit back so that bar is just below scapula/shoulder blades. Take hands and head back slowly.

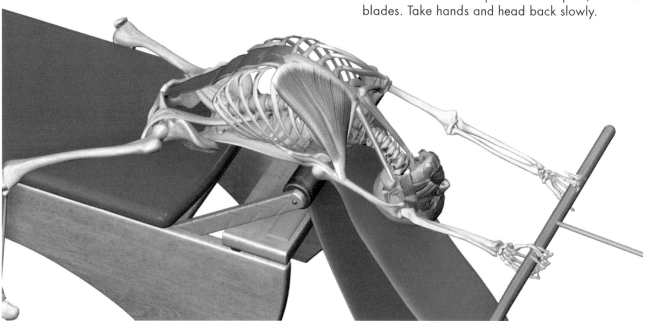

How to contract

Press hands and thighs up toward ceiling.

How to restretch

Allow pelvis, legs and arms to drop/flop.
Partner can pull arms downward and alternately pull one side more.

What to watch out for:

- Unnecessary tension in arms, neck, stomach.
- Dizziness.

Variation

Change sitting position so that different parts of the spine contact the bar. Change the direction of pull too, so that it varies from backwards to downwards depending on comfort/tolerance.

Lateral Flexion

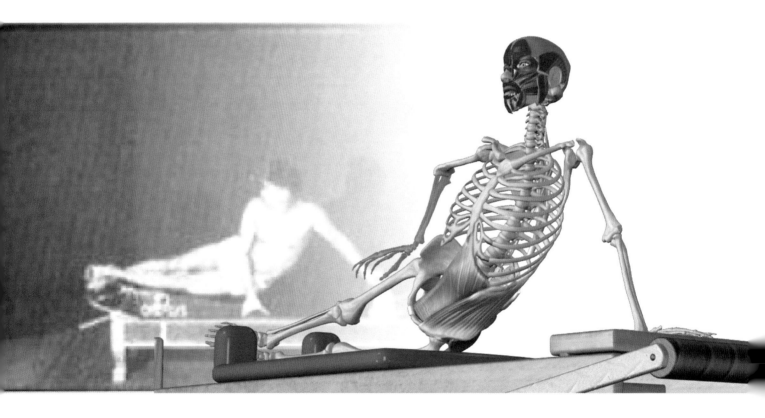

The Mermaid

- **Standard:** Beginner/Intermediate • **Spring Tension:** Light - Medium
- **Muscle Emphasis:** Oblique abdominals, quadratus lumborum, intercostals, abductors

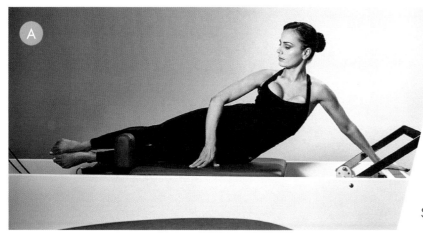

A & B. How to stretch

Slide carriage out and sit in center.
Place top leg/foot on top of bottom
leg/foot. Align feet, hips, hand,
ensure top hip above bottom hip.
Slide carriage in to POT to find stretch.

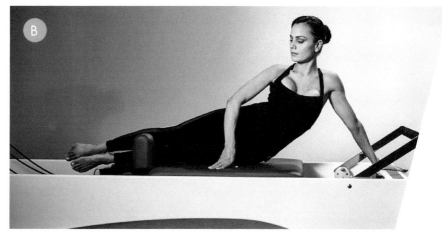

B. How to contract

Press hands and feet
down into floor.

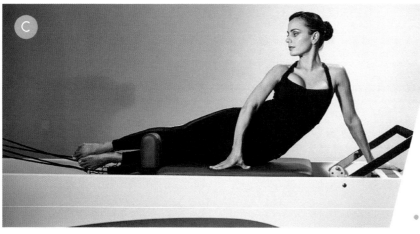

C. How to restretch

Slide carriage in further.
Deepen inhalations as
much as possible.

What to watch out for:

- Not aligning top hip with feet.

Variations

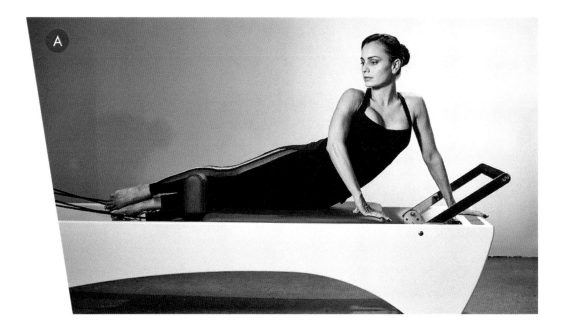

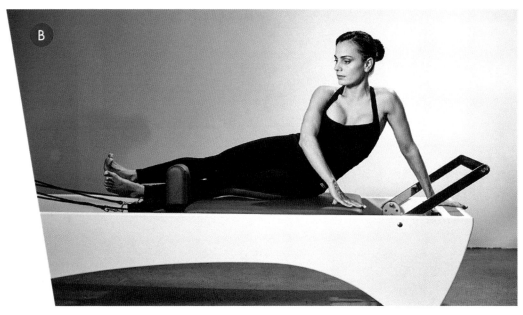

Roll top hip forward (A) and backward (B)
to shift stretch around.

As the carriage slides in, the spine is bent further sideways. The internal obliques will stretch along with the hip abductors gluteus medius and minimus, the quadatus lumborum and half of the erector spinae group.

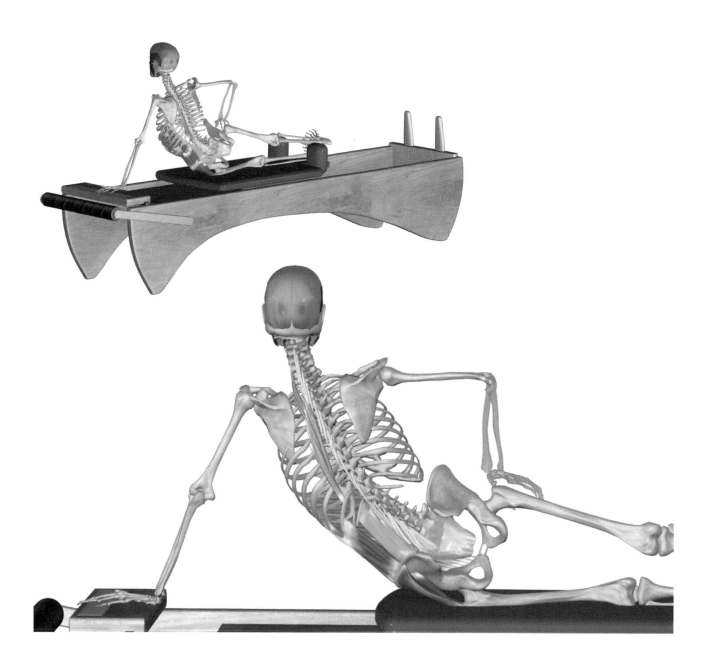

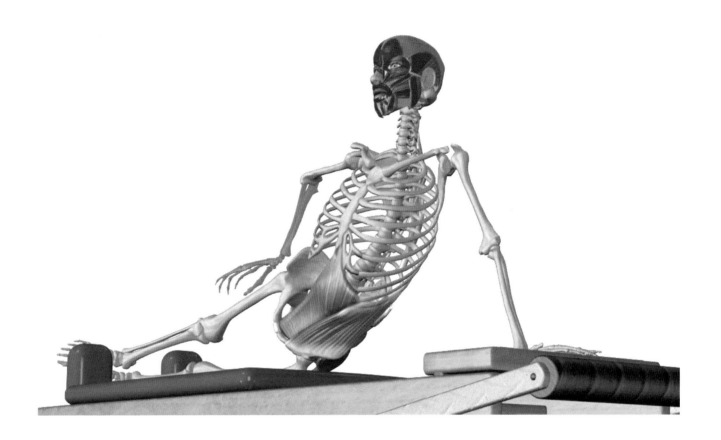

The internal obliques, lying "deep" to or underneath the external obliques, will also be stretched as you explore different hip angles.

Deep inhalations will increase the stretch. As the diaphragm descends, it will push the non-compressible abdominal content out towards the obliques, stretching them further.

The Seated Side Bend

- **Standard:** Beginner/Intermediate • **Spring Tension:** Light - Medium
- **Muscle Emphasis:** Oblique abdominals, quadratus lumborum, intercostals, latissimus dorsi, erector spine one side, long head of triceps

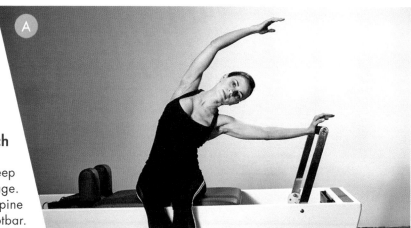

A. How to stretch

Push carriage out and keep both sit bones on carriage. Reach arm over and bend spine and rib cage away from footbar.

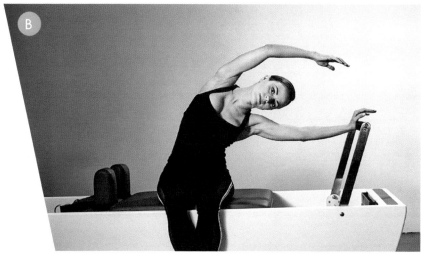

A. How to contract

Imagine pressing outside shoulder away from footbar.

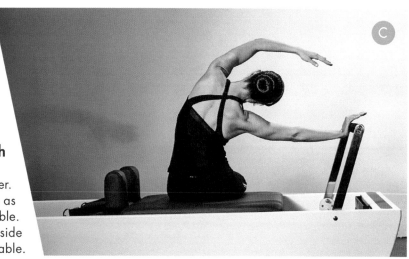

B & C. How to restretch

Slide carriage out a little further. Deepen inhalations as much as possible. Bend spine and head to side as much as is comfortable.

Variations

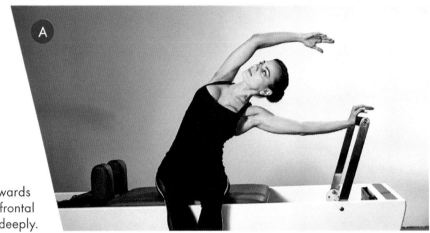

(A) Roll top shoulder backwards to move the stretch to the frontal abdominal area. Inhale deeply.

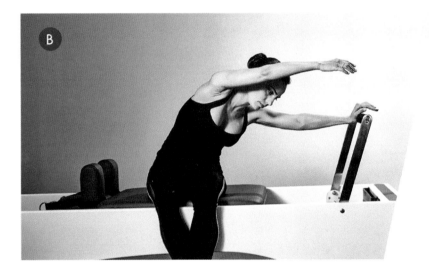

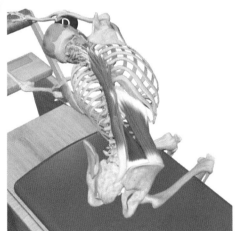

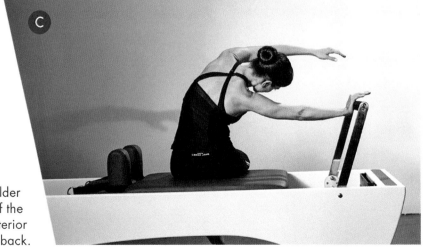

(B, C & D) Roll top shoulder forward to move the locus of the stretch to the posterior of the lower back.

Partner Assists

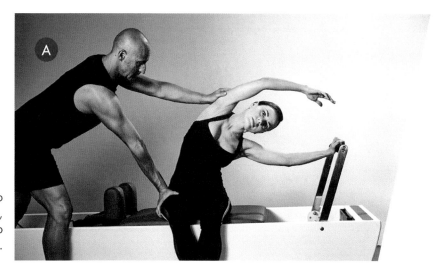

(A) Partner leans weight onto upper thigh to anchor pelvis, while pressing lightly into armpit to increase sidebend.

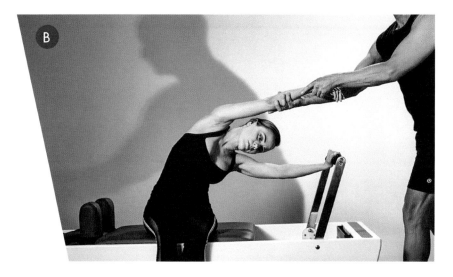

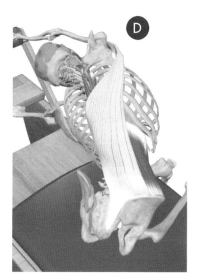

(B & D) Partner takes forearm and hand and pulls lightly to increase side bend and Latissimus Dorsi stretch.

(C) Partner changes position so as to change line of pull and increase rotation. This moves the stretch further toward posterior muscles of lower back. See image on previous page.

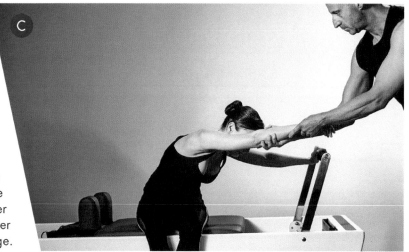

The Kneeling Banana

- **Standard:** Intermediate • **Spring Tension:** Medium
- **Muscle Emphasis:** Oblique abdominals, quadratus lumborum, intercostals, latissimus dorsi, abductors of hip

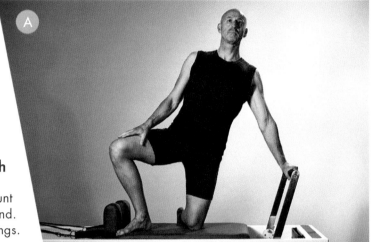

A & B. How to stretch

Push carriage out a short amount and align foot, knee and hand. Lower hips toward springs.

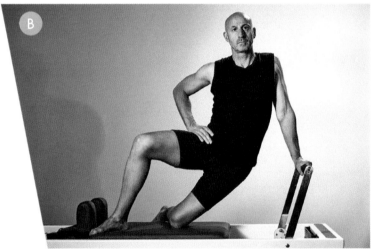

B. How to contract

Press hips up into top hand.

C. How to restretch

Lower hips further. Deepen inhalations as much as possible.

What to watch for

- Pushing carriage out too far.
- Not lowering hips enough.
- Not aligning body as described above.

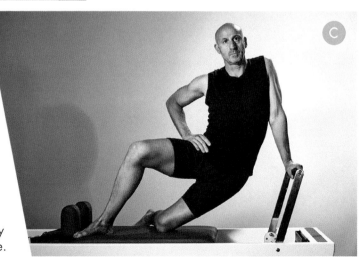

Variations

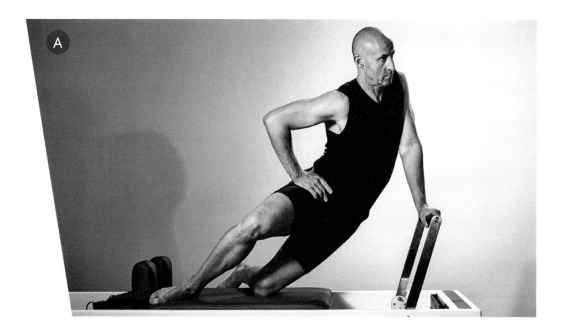

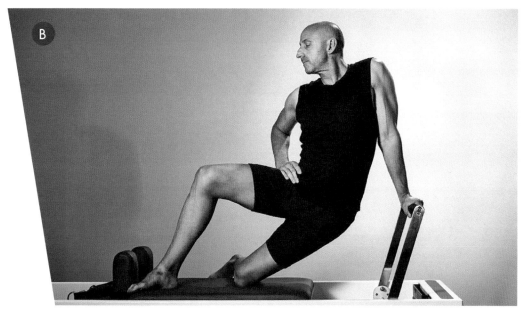

(A) Roll top hip forward (B) and backward to shift stretch around.

The Standing Banana

- **Standard:** Intermediate /Advanced • **Spring Tension:** Medium
- **Muscle Emphasis:** Oblique abdominals, quadratus lumborum, intercostals, latissimus dorsi, abductors of hip

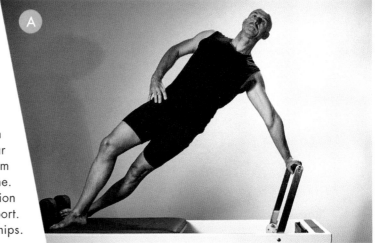

A. How to stretch

Push carriage away, straighten botton leg. Align hand on footbar with bottom hip and foot. Support arm at roughly 90 degrees to spine.
B. Shift top foot to position shown for greater support.
C. Lower hips.

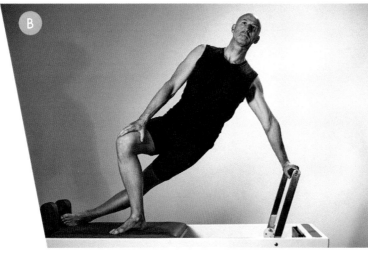

C. How to contract

Press hips up.

C. How to restretch

Lower hips further. Deepen inhalations as much as possible.

What to watch for

- Pushing carriage out too far.
- Not lowering hips enough.
- Not aligning body as described above.

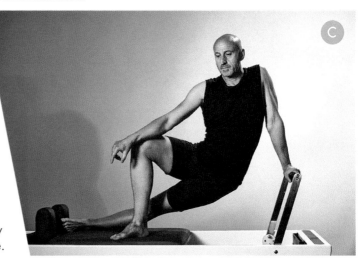

Variations

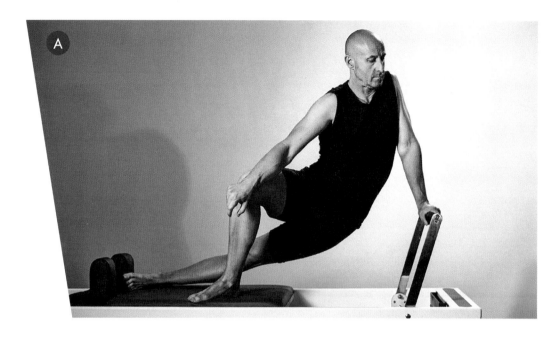

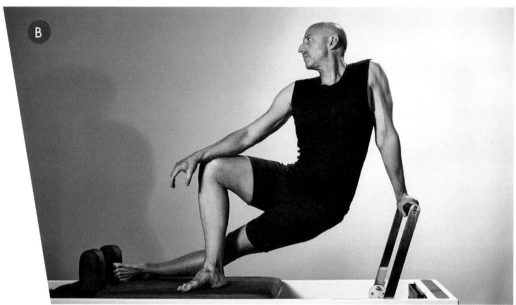

(A) Roll top hip forward (B) and backward to shift stretch around.

Chapter Seven

Arms & Shoulders

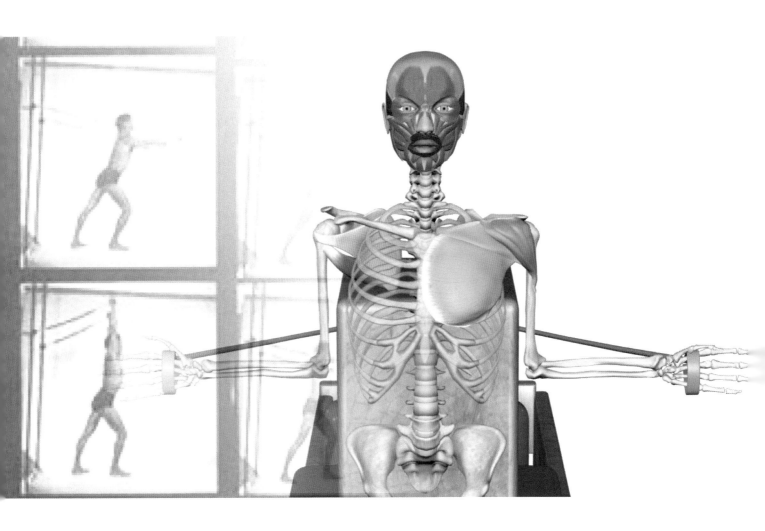

The Wrist Flexors

- Standard: Any • Spring Tension: no springs
- Muscle Emphasis: All wrist flexors

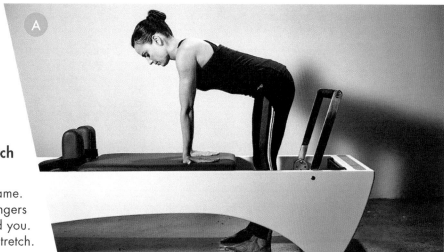

A. How to stretch

Stand inside reformer frame.
Place palms onto carriage with fingers
facing toward you.
Slide carriage out to find stretch.

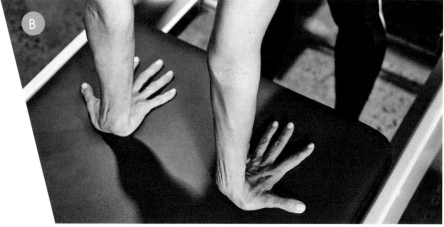

A & B. How to contract

Press palms and fingers down
into carriage.

C. How to restretch

Slide carraige away further.

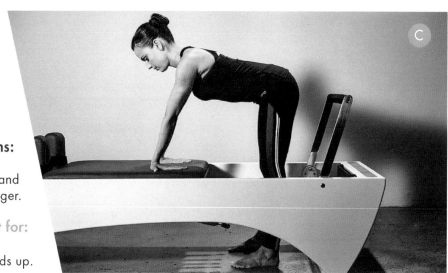

Variations:

Shift weight back and
around above each finger.

What to watch out for:

- Lifting palms of hands up.

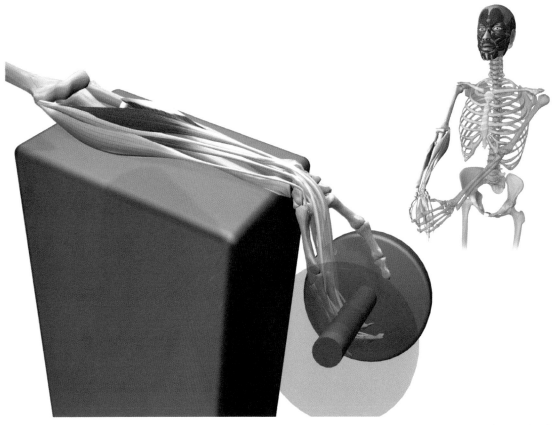

The forearm has both primary and secondary muscles that flex the wrist. You can see some of them attaching just above the inside of the elbow, or medial epicondyle, and running across the wrist as they become tendinous. This region is known as the carpal tunnel, where nine flexor tendons pass though this small compartment. Stretching will help to prevent carpel tunnel syndrome.

The Wrist Extensors

- **Standard:** Any • **Spring Tension:** no springs
- **Muscle Emphasis:** All wrist extensors

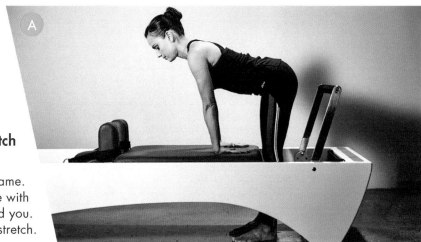

A. How to stretch

Stand inside reformer frame.
Place back of hands onto carriage with
fingers facing toward you.
Slide carriage out to find stretch.

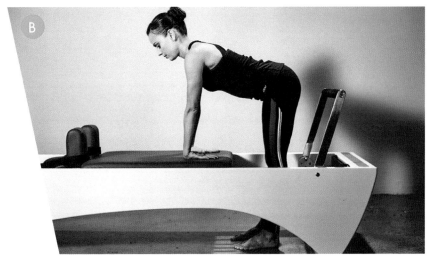

B. How to contract

Press back of hands and
fingers down into carriage.

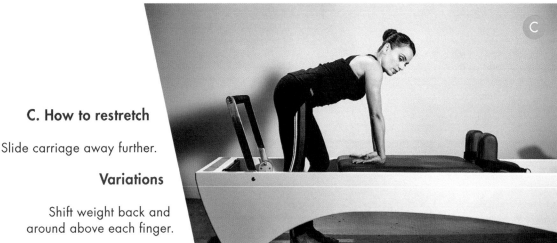

C. How to restretch

Slide carriage away further.

Variations

Shift weight back and
around above each finger.

The Lats

- **Standard:** Any • **Spring Tension:** Light to Medium
- **Muscle Emphasis:** Latissimus dorsi, oblique abdominals, quadratus lumborum, rotator cuff, log head triceps, erector spinae

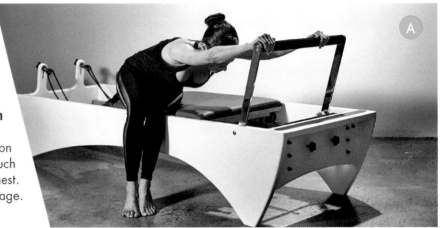

A. How to stretch

Sit on side of carriage with hands on footbar. Press carriage away as much as possible and lower chest. Lean shoulders away from carriage.

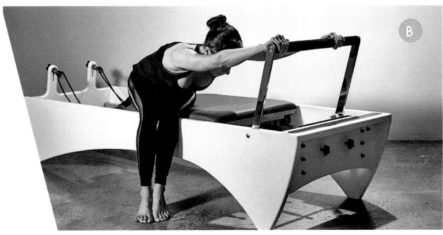

B. How to contract

Pull on footbar with outside hand; i.e. hand closest to end of footbar.

B & C. How to restretch

Slide carriage away further Lean shoulders further to side. Press inside hand firmly into foot bar.

C. Variations

Raise/lift outside shoulder and lower inside shoulder. Continue to lean to side.

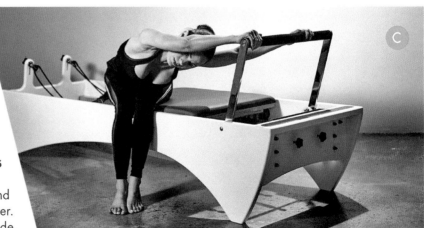

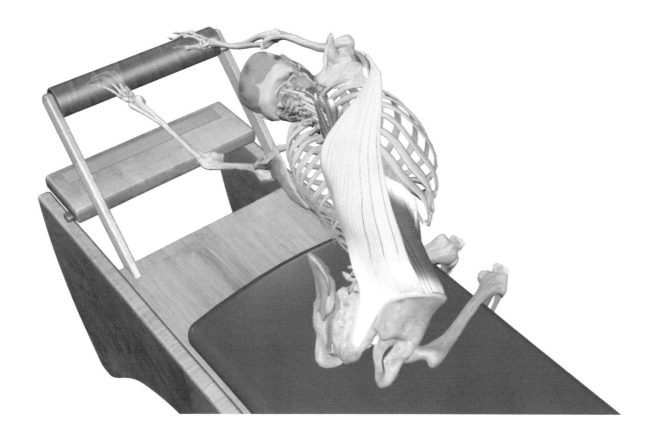

The Latissimus Dorsi and its little helper, Teres Major, are stretched strongly as you lean away from the reformer carriage. If you can keep both sit bones on the carriage, your Internal Obliques will be stretched more strongly too.

One half of the erector spinae are stretched,
Along with the quadratus lumborum and teres major.

Underneath, or "deep" to the erector spinae, you can see the   group stretching also. This muscle group stabilizes the joints of the spine.

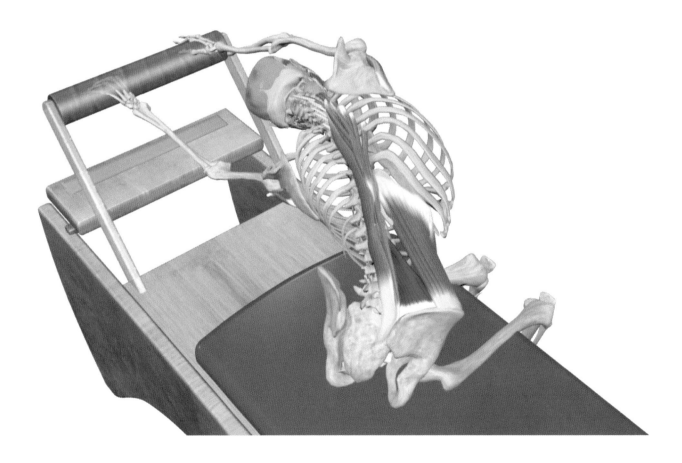

Internal Shoulder Rotators

- **Standard:** Any • **Spring Tension:** Medium to Heavy
- **Muscle Emphasis:** Teres major, subscapularis, anterior deltoid, clavicular portion of pectoralis major

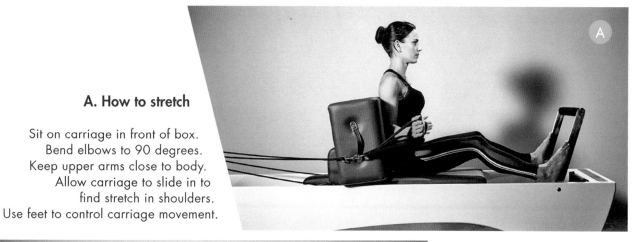

A. How to stretch

Sit on carriage in front of box.
Bend elbows to 90 degrees.
Keep upper arms close to body.
Allow carriage to slide in to
find stretch in shoulders.
Use feet to control carriage movement.

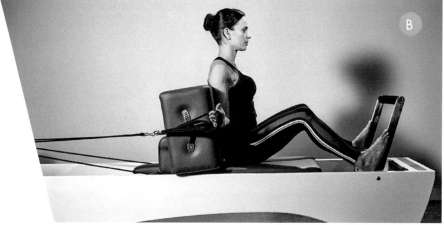

A. How to contract

Press hands into straps in
clapping motion.

B. How to restretch

Slide carriage further in.
Control movement with legs.

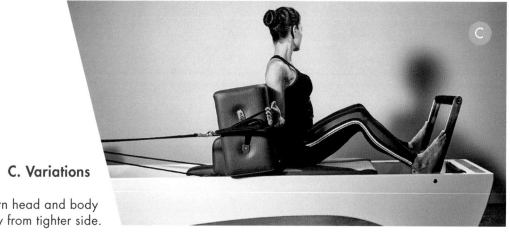

C. Variations

Carefully turn head and body
away from tighter side.

No Box?

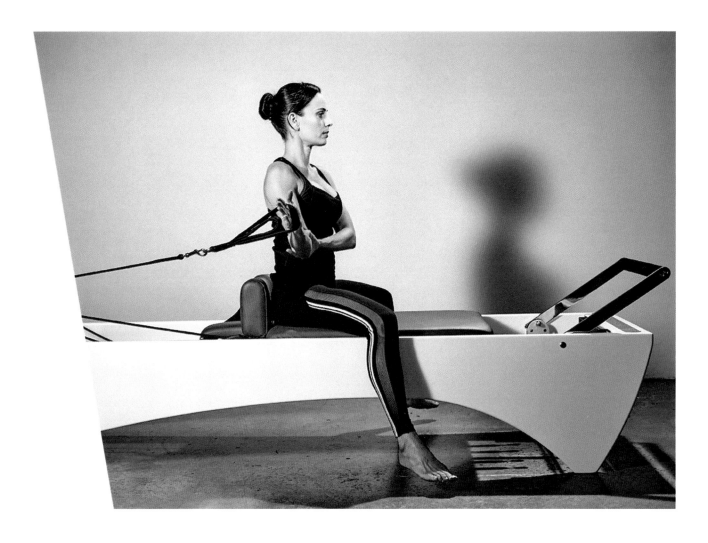

Reach around and hold your elbow with one hand and keep it from moving. Allow the carriage to slide in as above.

The subscapularis and teres major are the two muscles stretched the most. The sensations may not be precise, but will stem from anywhere round the shoulder joint.

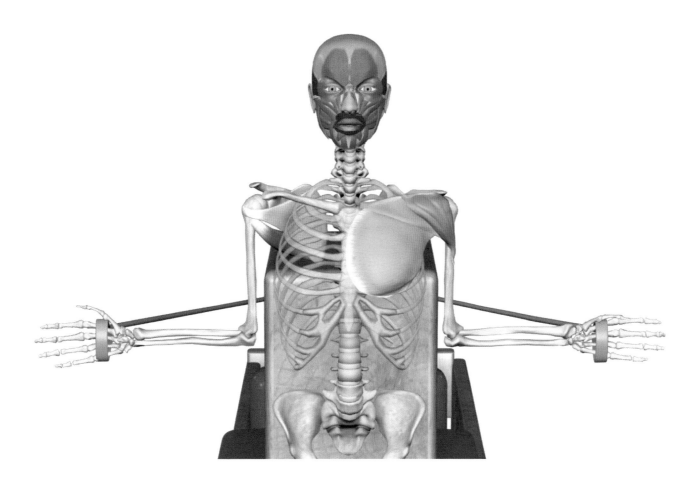

If you are tight, the pectoralis major – in particular its costal fibers – may stretch, as well as the anterior deltoid.

External Shoulder Rotators

- **Standard:** Any • **Spring Tension:** Medium to Heavy
- **Muscle Emphasis:** Infraspinatus, teres minor, posterior deltoid

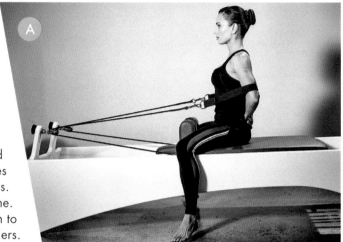

A & B. How to stretch

Sit on carriage with straps/ropes crossed over. Bend elbows to 90 degrees with straps just above elbows. Hands on lower lumbar spine. Allow carriage to slide in to find stretch in shoulders.

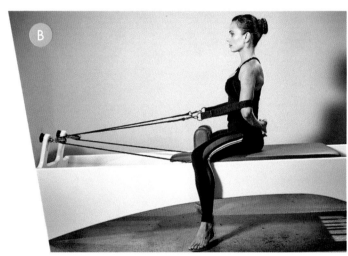

B. How to contract

Press hands into lower back.

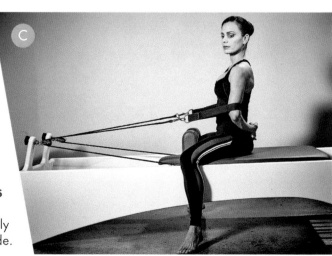

C. How to restretch

Slide carriage further in. Control movement with legs.

Variations

Turn body and head carefully toward tighter side.

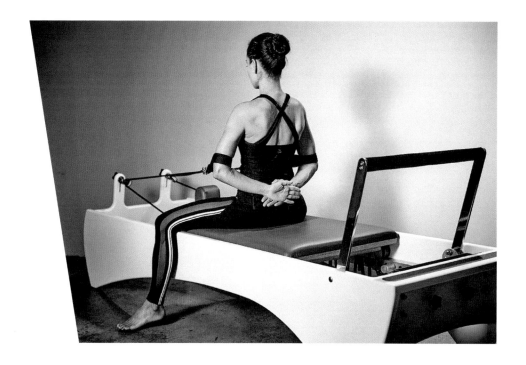

Hold the shoulder blades in place; i.e. Don't permit them to slide away from each other or "protract". This is done by contracting the trapezius and rhomboid muscles.

If you do this effectively, the infraspinatus, teres minor and posterior deltoid will stretch.

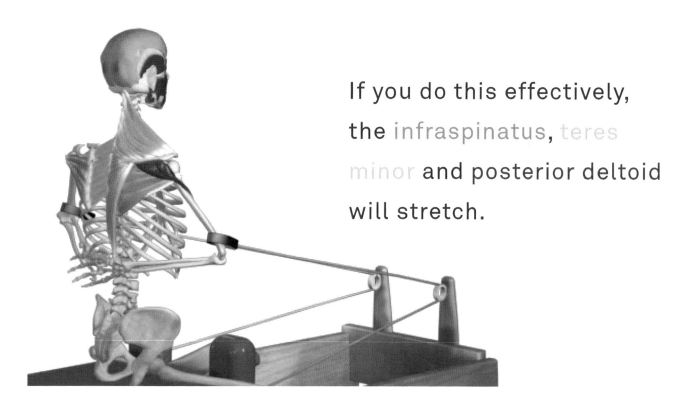

Pec Major

- **Standard:** Any • **Spring Tension:** Medium
- **Muscle Emphasis:** Pectoralis major, pectoralis minor, anterior deltoid

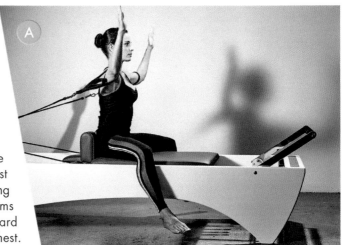

A & B. How to stretch

Sit as pictured, with straps either just above or just below elbow. Raise elbows to at least shoulder height (you can explore having elbows at different heights). Keep forearms vertical. Allow carriage to creep in toward resting position to POT. Lift chest.

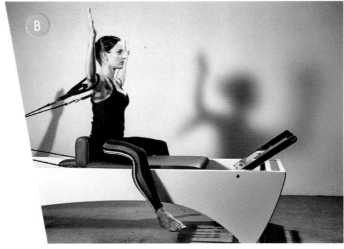

B. How to contract

Press forearms and elbows toward each other in clapping motion.

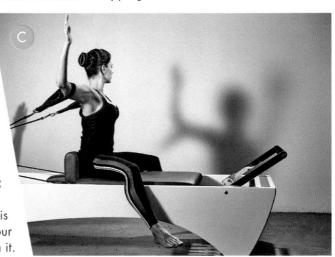

C. How to restretch

Allow carriage to slide in further toward resting position.

C. Variations:

If you have one side that is particularly tight, turn your head and chest away from it.

Alternate Position

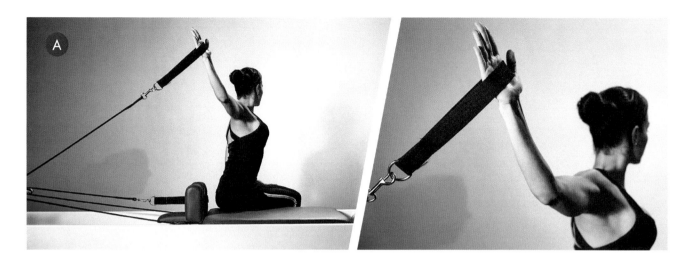

Sit on one side of the reformer. Place strap into opposite hand. Raise arm, sit tall and lean chest away from arm. Rotate chest/head away from arm for greater effect. Contract by pulling on strap.
Restretch by repeating instructions above.

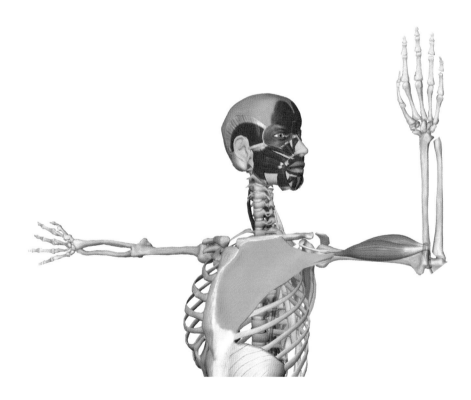

Pectoralis Minor

- **Standard:** Any • **Spring Tension:** Medium
- **Muscle Emphasis:** Pectoralis major, pectoralis minor, anterior deltoid, biceps brachii

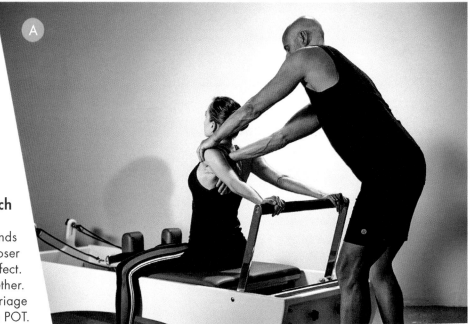

A. How to stretch

Sit as pictured, and place hands on footbar. Place hands closer together for stronger effect. Draw shoulder blades together. Lift chest and slide carriage away slowly to POT.

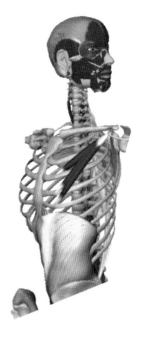

How to contract

Press hands down into footbar.

How to restretch

Lift chest. Slide carriage away further.

What to watch out for:

- Flexing/rounding chest/thorax.
- Allowing shoulders to round/ protracting scapula.
- Internally rotating arms.

Variations

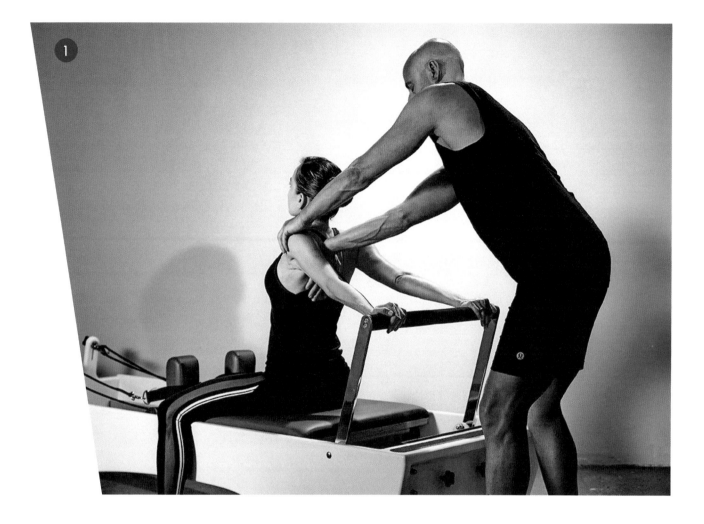

Turn head and chest away from tight side.

If you have a partner available, have them place one hand on your shoulder blade and press it firmly onto your rib cage. Have them place the other hand on the front of your shoulder and draw the shoulder backwards. Follow other instructions.

Deltoid

- **Standard**: Any • **Spring Tension**: Heavy
- **Muscle Emphasis**: Deltoid, rhomboids, middle trapezius

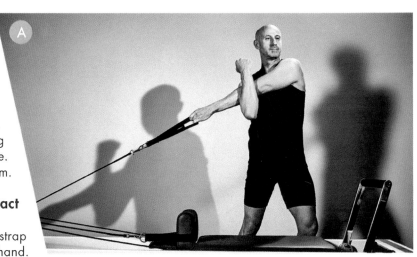

A. How to stretch

Stand or sit as pictured.
Lean away from strap, ensuring
carriage does not move.
Pull arm onto chest with free arm.

A. How to contract

Attempt to swing arm holding strap
away from chest as if to hit a backhand.

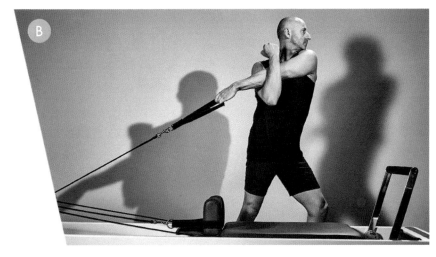

B. How to restretch

Lift chest and lean further
away from strap. Rotate/turn
chest away from strap.

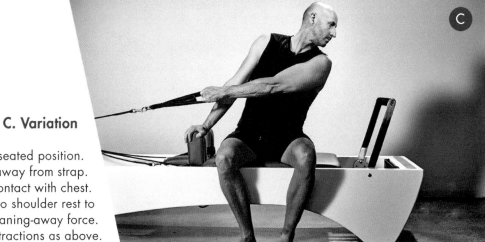

C. Variation

Try seated position.
Lean away from strap.
Keep arm in contact with chest.
Press free hand into shoulder rest to
increase leaning-away force.
Contractions as above.

Supraspinatus

- **Standard:** Any • **Spring Tension:** Heavy
- **Muscle Emphasis:** Supraspinatus, deltoid

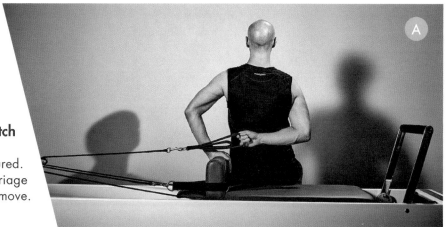

A & B. How to stretch

Stand or sit as pictured. Lean away from strap ensuring carriage does not move.

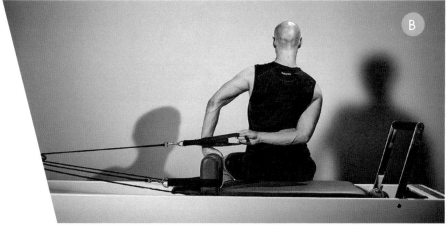

B. How to contract

Attempt to pull elbow away from body.

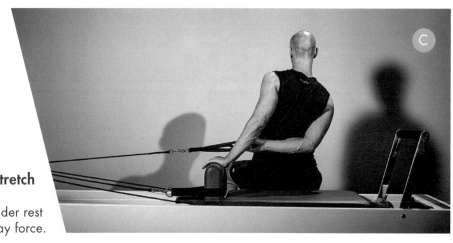

B & C. How to restretch

Press free hand into shoulder rest to increase leaning-away force.

Biceps Brachii

- **Standard:** Any • **Spring Tension:** Heavy
- **Muscle Emphasis:** Biceps brachii, brachialis, anterior deltoid

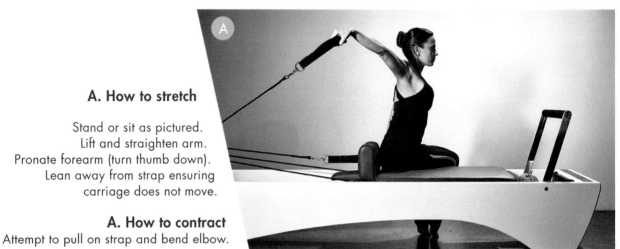

A. How to stretch

Stand or sit as pictured.
Lift and straighten arm.
Pronate forearm (turn thumb down).
Lean away from strap ensuring
carriage does not move.

A. How to contract

Attempt to pull on strap and bend elbow.

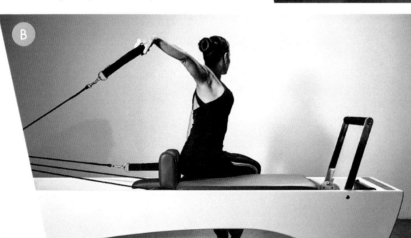

B. How to restretch

Lean further from strap.
Rotate chest away from arm.

C. What to watch for

- Internally rotating
shoulder of stretching arm.
- Dropping stretching arm.
- Allowing carriage to move.
Photo C shows how to
maintain good form.

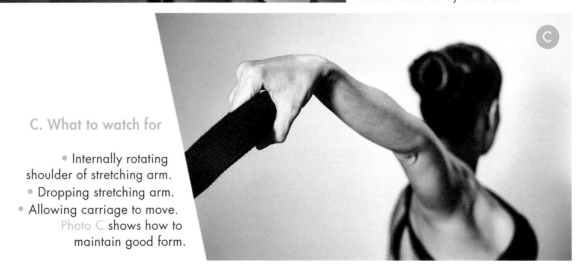

Chapter Eight

The Splits

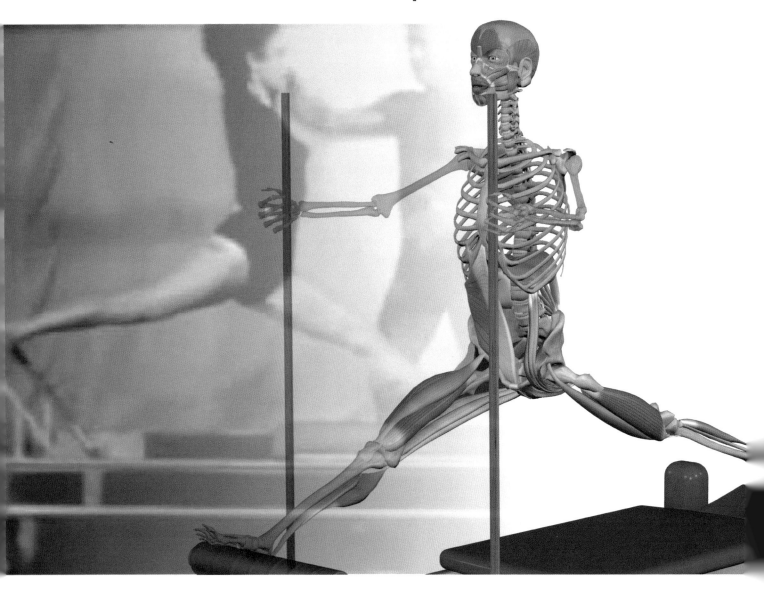

The "True Front Splits"

- **Standard:** Advanced • **Spring Tension:** Medium
- **Muscle Emphasis:** All hip flexors rear leg, hamstrings & calves front leg

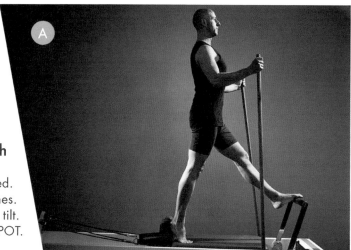

A & B. How to stretch

Stand on reformer as pictured.
Ensure hips are square at all times.
Maintain neutral or posterior pelvic tilt.
Lower hips to POT.

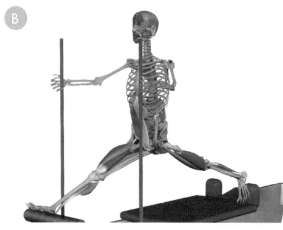

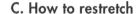

B. How to contract

Press both feet down.

C. How to restretch

Lower hips further.
Lift chest.

What to watch out for:

- Externally rotating rear leg.
  - Anterior pelvic tilt.
  - Leaning trunk forward
    toward hip flexion.

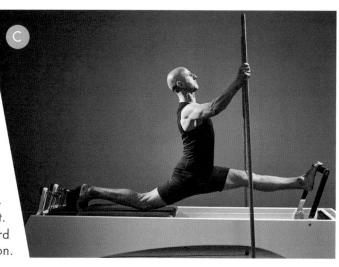

The psoas major attaches from as high up as the 12th thoracic vertebrae. Inside the pelvis it joins with the illiacus to wrap around the front of the pelvis and insert onto the lesser trochanter of the femur. The rectus femoris is also under considerable stretch.

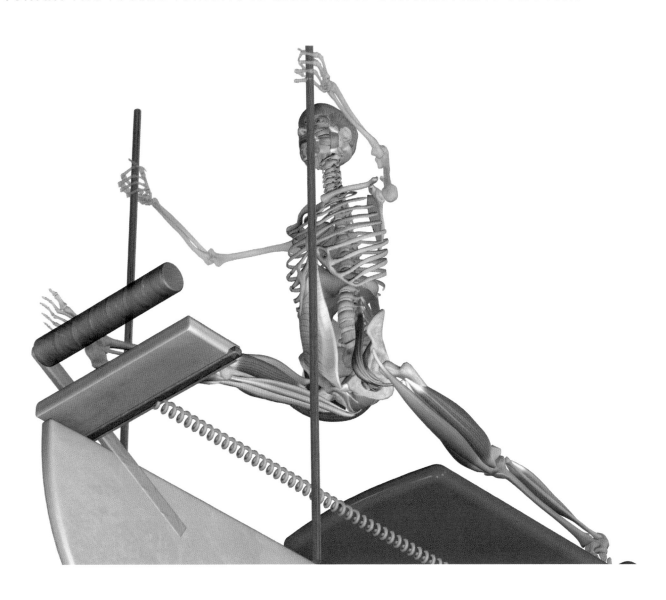

If the pelvis is maintained in the correct neutral position, the hamstrings will be stretched strongly. Their origins are underneath the pelvis and located posteriorly.

Variation

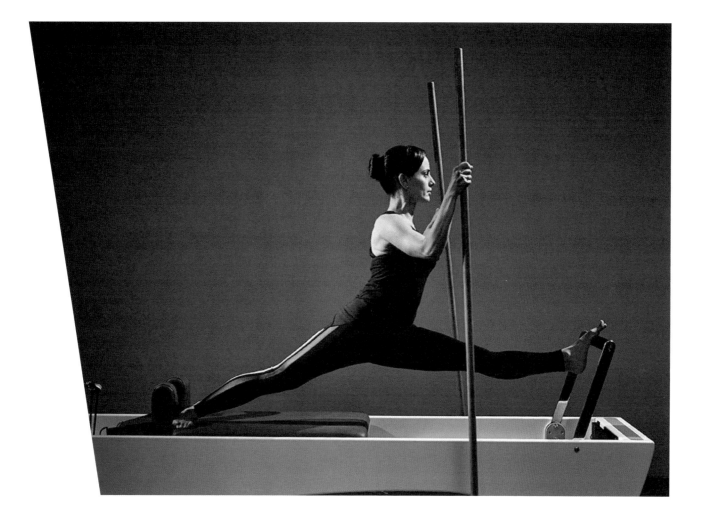

The traditional "dancers front split" has the rear leg externally rotated.

In addition, the low back is hyperextended. This enables the ligaments of the hip to be slackened and a fuller, more complete looking split position to be achieved. The stretch in the rear leg diminishes in the hip flexors and is more focused on the adductors.

 For a fuller discussion of the front splits, refer to our online workshop titled "The Splits", or to "Innovations in Pilates, Therapeutic Muscle Stretching on the Pilates Reformer".

The Bent Leg Front Splits

• **Standard:** Advanced • **Spring Tension:** Medium
• **Muscle Emphasis:** All hip flexors rear leg, hamstrings, gluteus maximus, adductor magnus front leg

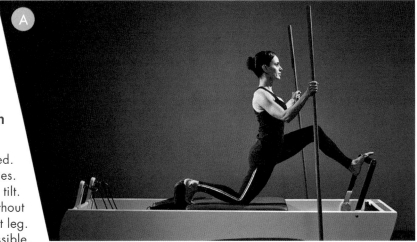

A & B. How to stretch

Kneel on reformer as pictured.
Ensure hips are square at all times.
Maintain neutral or posterior pelvic tilt.
Lower hips to POT, without
straightening front leg.
Press back leg back as far as possible.

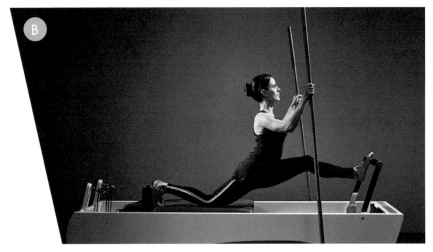

B. How to contract

Press both feet down.

C. How to restretch

Lift rear knee off carriage a fraction and try to straighten it.
Then try to straighten front leg
(*not shown*). Lift chest.

What to watch out for:

• Externally rotating rear leg.
• Lifting hip along with rear knee.

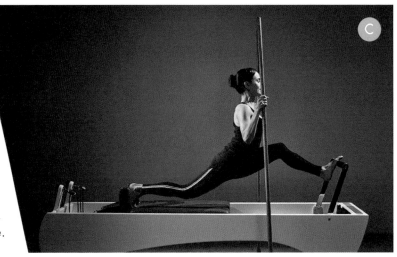

The Side Splits

- **Standard:** Advanced • **Spring Tension:** Medium
- **Muscle Emphasis:** All adductors, medial hanstrings

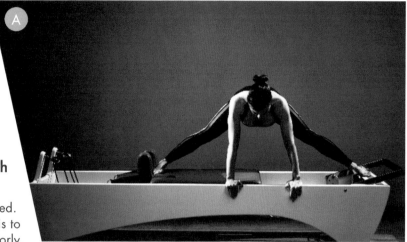

A & B. How to stretch

Stand on reformer as pictured. Lower hips to POT, allow pelvis to rotate forward/anteriorly.

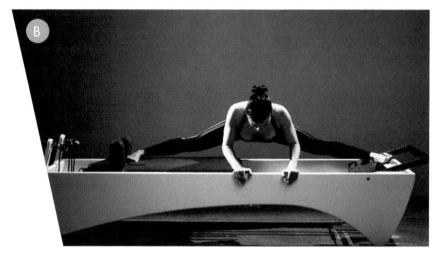

B. How to contract

Press both feet down. Tighten quadriceps.

C. How to restretch

Press carriage away with abductors. Lower hips. Take weight onto arms. Allow low back to hyperextend.

What to watch out for:

- Pain in knee or hip joints.

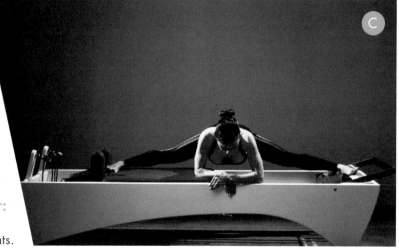

Variations:
To focus on one leg at a time

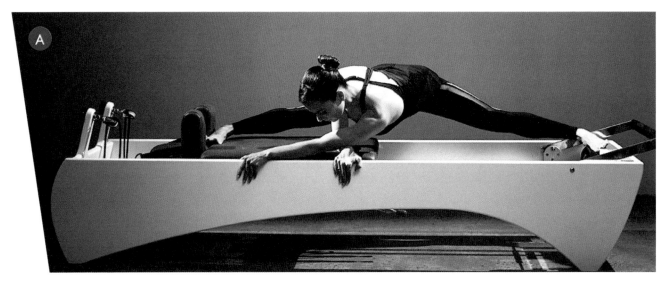

Turn chest and shoulders in one direction...

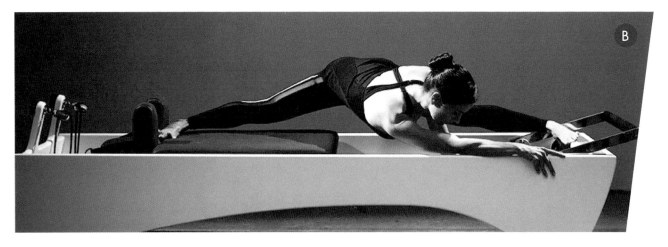

... and then the other.

Bibliography

Ahearn, G. 2008. *General Anatomy: Principles and Applications*. McGraw Hill. Australia

Alter, MJ. 1996. *Science of Flexibility*. Human Kinetics. Australia.

Armiger, P. 2010. Stretching for functional Flexibility. Lippincott Wiliams & Wilkins. USA.

Chaitow, L. 1988. *Soft Tissue Manipulation*. Healing Arts Press. Rochester, Vermont.

Coulter, HD. 2002. *Anatomy of Hatha Yoga*. Body and Breath. Honesdale, USA.

Frederick, A, and Frederick, C. 2006. *Stretch to Win*. Human Kinetics. Australia.

Grilley, P. 2004. *Anatomy for Yoga*. http://www.pranamaya.com

Jerome, J. 1987. *Fitness Stretching*. Breakaway Books. NY.

Juhan, D. 1987. *Job's Body*. Station Hill Press. NY.

Kapandji, LA. 1974. *The Physiology of the Joints*. Volumes 1–3. Churchill Livingstone. Edinburgh.

Kendall, HO. 1971. *Muscles, Testing and Function*. 2nd Edition. Williams and Wilkins. Baltimore.

Knott, M, & Voss, DE. 1968. *Proprioceptive Neuromuscular Facilitation*. Harper and Row. NY.

Kurtz, T. 1994. *Stretching Scientifically*. Stadion Publishing. USA.

Lederman, A. 2014. *Therapeutic Stretching*. Human Kinetics. Australia.

Long, R. 2005. *The Key Muscles of Hatha Yoga*. Bhandhayoga Publications. USA.

Long, R. 2008. *The Key Poses of Hatha Yoga*. Bhandhayoga Publications. USA.

McAtee, RE. 2007. *Facilitated Stretching*. Human Kinetics. Australia.

Myers, TW. 2009. *Anatomy Trains*. Churchill Livingstone. Sydney.

Neuman, DA. 2002. *Kinesiology of the Musculoskeletal System*. Mosby. USA.

Norris, C. 2004. *The Complete Guide to Stretching*. A & C Black Publishers. London.

Pilates, J. 1934. *Your Health.* Presentation Dynamics. Copywrited and reprinted 1988. USA.

Pilates, J. 1945. *Pilates' Return to Life through Contrology*. Presentation Dynamics. Copywrited and reprinted 1998. USA.

Richardson, JHH. 1999. *Therapeutic Exercise for Spinal Segmental Stabilization in Low Back Pain*. Churchill Livingstone. Sydney.

Sahrmann, SA. 2002. *Diagnosis and Treatment of Movement Impairment Syndromes*. Mosby. USA.

Tsatsouline, P. 2001. *Relax into Stretch*. Dragon Door Publications. USA.

Thompson, F. 1994. *Manual of Structural Kinesiology*. Mosby. Sydney.

Ylinen, J. 2008. *Stretching Therapy*. Churchill Livingstone. Sydney

Thank You!

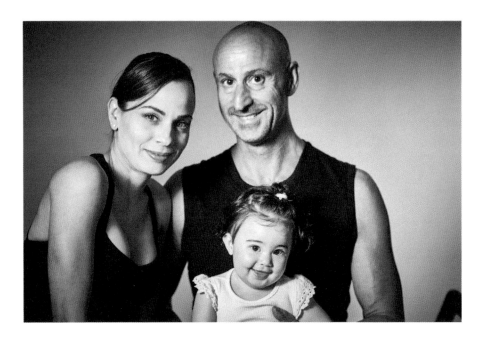

Dear Readers,

Thank you again for continuing your quest for health with us.

Please keep in touch with us at www.innovationsinpilates.com or https://www.facebook.com/Innovations-in-Pilates-519771898058940/timeline/

As always, stay loose!

Warm regards from Anthony, Kenyi and Grace.

Made in the USA
Columbia, SC
24 January 2018